A NATURAL CURE FOR CANCER

As Told By Survivors

How Cancer is Healed with Shark Cartilage, Wheat Grass Juice, Macrobiotics, Germanium, and Other Natural Remedies

D. INGEBRITSON

RDINGE, LLC
Fort Worth, TX

Organizations, companies and individuals mentioned in the book may not necessarily agree with views expressed by the author. Brand-names herein are protected by law.

First Edition: March, 2003
Copyright © 2003 by D. Ingebritson
All rights reserved.

Cover Design: Bookcovers. com
Editing: Jan Gary Communications, Arlington, TX

Publisher's Cataloging-in-Publication
(Provided by Quality Books, Inc.)

Ingebritson, D.
    A natural cure for cancer : as told by survivors :
how cancer is healed with shark cartilage, wheat grass
juice, macrobiotics, germanium and other natural
remedies / D. Ingebritson. – 1 st ed.
    p. cm.
    ISBN 0-615-12157-8

    1. Cancer–Alternative treatment. 2. Cancer–Diet
therapy. I. Title.

RC271.A62154 2003   616.99´406
                             QBI03-200183

Published by: RDINGE LC
P.O. Box 16354
Fort Worth, TX 76162 Fax: 817-292-2576

Printed in the United States of America

"I have no special talents. I am only passionately curious."
-Albert Einstein

READ THIS CAREFULLY!

This book is based on my personal experiences and beliefs. I have no medical training and in no way am I providing medical advice. What is included is for educational purposes only. Should you have health problems, consult with caring and qualified health professionals. Don't attempt anything on your own. Some of what is mentioned could cause serious injury or even death. I disclaim all liability resulting from the use of information in the book – always seek proper medical approval. In addition, any consultation provided by telephone will be limited to diets, relaxation, yoga, motivation, support and lifestyle – *nothing more than opinions*. See back of the book for details.

—Dan Ingebritson

TABLE OF CONTENTS

Preface 7
Introduction: Can This Be Happening to Me? 9
My experience with early stage melanoma skin cancer

Chapters
1. Cancer - A Simple View 17
Doctors who treat cancer may say I am mistaken
2. Treatments for Cancer 21
Surgery, radiation and chemotherapy – the truth
3. Causes of Cancer 25
What is believed
4. The Cold Realities of Cancer 29
Cancer is relentless
5. Food and Cancer 35
*processed foods * fish and meats * grains * vegetables
and fruits * water * vitamins and supplements *
herbs * teas * honey * nuts*
6. Lifestyle to Prevent Cancer 51
*healthy eating habits * we live in a dangerous world
* personal care for the body * exercise * sleep * the
skin * health problems * stress. People who do not
develop cancer; people who do get cancer.*
7. Diagnosed with Cancer 67
Making decisions

8.Alternative Therapies 71

*Iscador * wheat grass juice * mushrooms * shark cartilage * macrobiotics * Essiac * the Moerman diet * Laetrile * IP6 * Entelev, Cancell or Cantron * Gerson Diet * the Tijuana connection * purge the parasite, cure the cancer * Poly-MVA * gene therapy * juice fasting *flaxseed oil * the power of the mind * the secret is oxygen * vaccines * enzyme therapy * hyperthermia * marijuana * Chinese remedies * germanium*

9. Healing Cancer Naturally 95

The common thread reveals the secret

10. Surviving Cancer 113

Yoga, meditation and deep relaxation

11. Afterthoughts 125

Resources 135

*Alternative organizations * Clinics * Books*

PREFACE

Cures and remedies. A cure restores good health and ends illness entirely. Remedies are treatments which attempt to cure or provide relief. Such therapy may treat symptoms and not causes. Only remedies are available for the treatment of cancer; a cure for cancer does not exist.

I have used "cure" in the title, because numerous men and women told me (personally, by telephone and through letters) that they rid cancer from their bodies with natural or alternative methods. Others in books and periodicals have made similar claims. I believe all of these individuals were sincere and truthful in communicating how they were cured. Nonetheless, I have determined there are distinct reasons for their surviving. And hopefully, I have provided an illuminating explanation.

Plus, I would like to acknowledge Nancy French, Ph.D., N.D., R.N., for her contribution, though any errors are my own.

Dan Ingebritson
March, 2003

INTRODUCTION:

Can This Be Happening to Me?

While outdoors on a summer day, I noticed that direct sunlight was irritating – mildly stinging – a very small mole on my right forearm. I wasn't too concerned; the mole was uniform in shape, and wasn't discolored or elevated. Previously, several small moles on my back had festered and come off on their own. I thought this mole might do the same. Another three weeks passed. It now appeared the mole had become slightly irregular in form and to a degree had turned redder. This made me uncomfortable, and I decided it should be taken off. When I was a teenager, a general practitioner removed a larger mole from my inner thigh. I didn't think there would be any problem.

I was mistaken, however. The local clinic of the Veterans Administration could not schedule an appointment with a dermatologist in reasonable time; and a doctor I knew, after learning the mole was more than three millimeters in diameter, wouldn't see me. He referred me to two dermatologists known to him. When contacting the offices for these physicians, I was told the first possible appointment was in two months. Calling other dermatologists in the telephone directory brought similar results. I now believed that my life could be in jeopardy. The ones working for these doctors knew a change in a mole can indicate melanoma cancer, but they chose to ignore my pleas.

That afternoon, I called the same dermatologists again – something had to be done. A cancellation occurred just when I telephoned one office, so luckily, I was allowed an early appointment. When the ordeal continued over my insurance coverage, I shouted into the phone, "*I will pay cash!*"

The next day, the mole was removed in a way to determine later what its underside was like. Three times the dermatologist told me he didn't think it was malignant, but that a pathologist must analyze it to be certain. I researched my health books. From what I read, melanoma moles are less ominous when they are shallow in the skin. Real trouble can result when they are situated on a vein or are deeper under the skin. Millimeters make a difference.

On Friday, there was a message from the dermatologist's office on my answering machine. I had not been sleeping well, and I wasn't thrilled by the tone of the nurse's voice on the recording. A quick call to the doctor's office brought unpleasant news that the mole was melanoma. The nurse added, "*It was at a very early stage. You don't have to take chemotherapy.*" This was a jolt and didn't cheer me at all. I was scheduled for an operation to learn if surrounding tissue might contain cancer. Not surprising to me now, the doctor was going on vacation and delaying the surgery was considered. I was insistent the procedure be done as soon as possible.

Several days later, I revisited the doctor's office. A

three-inch incision was made directly over where the mole had been. The skin was peeled back and tissue samples were taken. This time the pathologist did not detect any malignancy. I felt better. I was told by the dermatologist that any future problem was extremely remote. Perhaps there was one chance in 95 of a recurrence. Regrettably, the few statistical graphs for melanoma that I've come across aren't nearly so optimistic.

I became aware of others who had a melanoma mole surgically taken off, and tissue samples, when scrutinized under slides, showed an absence of cancer. Sometime later, however, melanoma reappeared as a tiny rubbery bump, exactly or near where the initial mole had been. Surgery removed this growth, and again, samples of tissue proved negative for cancer. Then, within a year or even much later, cancerous tumors were discovered throughout their body – in the lymph nodes, liver and lungs. These tumors were the result of a few malignant cells which had somehow remained, then migrated or entered the bloodstream.

If cancer had been uncovered with the probe performed on my arm, I believed that chemotherapy would be the appropriate treatment. I could endure this if necessary, but I soon discovered chemotherapy was decidedly worthless in the treatment of melanoma. In truth, any therapy is ineffective; the majority with advanced melanoma are dead within a couple of years.

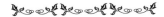

For much of my adult life I had been a vegetarian. I frequented health food stores weekly, seeking to gain more energy and better health with every product recommended. I practiced yoga daily and had believed that I was invulnerable to cancer, even skin cancer. I had knowledge of countless health remedies. But with this unsettling event, I knew I must obtain better health, acquire greater knowledge of cancer, and learn more about alternative remedies. My life could depend upon this.

What first came to mind was recalling a woman I had met in 1977 when I lived in Australia. Margaret Fenzel (of Russian descent and an immigrant to Australia) at the time had said to me that five years earlier three oncologists (cancer specialists) had told her she was terminal with cancer and that nothing could be done. Margaret screamed into the face of one doctor, "*I refuse to die!*" She began planting kernels of wheat in small wooden boxes and cutting the grass when it grew six inches high. Each afternoon, she sat quietly by herself and drank a large glass of **wheat grass juice**. I once shared a glass with her. I had not kept up with her since our earlier meeting, but I telephoned friends in Australia who knew her. They told me that she had died in 2000 – from heart failure, not cancer. Supposedly, her recent doctors were taken aback when informed of her earlier cancer incident and method for surviving.

I continued with my research. At the book section of a health food store, I rediscovered *Eat Right 4 Your Type,* by Peter J. D'Adamo, N.D. (naturopathic physician). I had rejected this book several years before because Dr. D'Adamo suggests those with Blood Type O should be meat eaters. I believed he was wrong, but, when reviewing his book this time, the explanations got my attention. Very reluctantly, I began following the plan and soon realized how well it works.

Bison, grass-fed cattle, sturgeon and sardines in spring water, along with spinach and figs have become regular parts of my diet. I conceded to the diet because health problems of a lifetime have ended. I have the energy, digestion, and more importantly, the understanding I had long sought.

Those with chronic health problems may benefit from another book by D'Adamo, *Live Right 4 Your Type*. I learned that I am a non-secretor for my blood type and knowing this revealed why I have had a lifetime of poor health. To learn your blood type or to know if you are a secretor or non-secretor, either be tested locally or obtain mail order self-test kits. Addresses for the kits are in his books.

At the Fort Worth Public Library, I checked out several books on cancer. One, *How to Fight Cancer & Win,* by William L. Fischer, offered hope. At Half Price Books™, I purchased two books, an old edition of *Options: The Alternative Cancer Therapy Book,* by Richard Walters, and *Cancer: Increasing Your Odds for Survival,* by David Bognar. I was familiar with many of the remedies detailed in these books and books read at the library – health food stores offer the same or similar literature and sell many of the products.

Ayurveda, the herbal medicine originating in India, was one of the remedies written about. I once followed it for a brief time. I consulted with Chinese herbal doctors when living in East Asia and was acquainted with most alternative treatments prescribed by them. These methods were discussed. Years before, I fasted (to forgo eating) in several ways and I tried juice diets. One book from the library described diets similar to these. Several books commented on **macrobiotics**, a natural foods diet brought to America from Japan six decades ago. I was on the macrobiotic diet for two years; and though helpful like other remedies or diets, it didn't resolve my health problems.

A number of books specified wheat grass juice as a remedy. I once grew it myself. If it was saving the lives of those with cancer, why wasn't this known? Something must be amiss – all of those drinking wheat grass juice probably are not surviving cancer. This must be true for all the other unheard-of remedies for cancer.

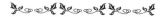

Dr. D'Adamo's *Eat Right 4 Your Type* (referred to as "The Blood Type Diet") proposes guidelines for meats, seafoods, oils, nuts, beans and legumes, vegetables, grains, fruits, spices, herbs and juices for each of the four blood types. Foods (or substances) listed as "Beneficial" for each blood type are said to be medicines; "Neutrals" are foods which supply energy and nutrients; "Avoid" foods are poisonous, even though a person may not realize it. For me, ingesting minuscule amounts of foods to avoid for Blood Type O cause stomach cramps shortly thereafter and fatigue within a day. Many times within the last 25 years, I eliminated individual foods (even grains) from my diet for a week or longer, but I could never discern the ones causing problems. Adhering to D'Adamo's plan does this perfectly for me. Having Blood Type O and being a non-secretor define who I am.

In each of his books, D'Adamo provides a noteworthy chapter on cancer, along with compelling advice for sustaining the immune system. His recommendations for Blood Type O, A, B and AB may help prevent cancer or be indispensable with treatment. Knowing your blood type and obtaining his books are necessary, in my opinion, to fully comprehend how cancer could be overcome. Public libraries and bookstores have the books.

CHAPTER ONE

Cancer — A Simple View

Published annually by the American Cancer Society, *Cancer Facts and Figures* provides valuable information. Books for specific cancers are also available from the Society. Tel: 800-ACS-2345. *Conversations About Cancer* by Michael Auerbach, M.D., is very informative and easy to read. *Cancer & Natural Medicine* by John Boik, is also suggested.

Existing cells generate new cells. In this way, bodies for both humans and animals are renewed. Occasionally, a cell gets the wrong instructions because of DNA damage, an aggravation, or for some other reason, and begets an abnormal cell which does not perform life-giving functions. (Several non-mainstream scientists argue that cells are not created in these ways.) Natural killer (NK) cells, white blood cells and the dendritic cells (octopus-like cells which control the immune system) guard the body against abnormal cells and other foreign objects. When potentially dangerous elements or unwanted cells are discovered, these cells of the immune system go on the attack, stick to them, and destroy or absorb them. This takes place in everyone's body at some time.

However, when certain abnormal cells elude detection and have the ability to fasten themselves within the body, they become clusters of cells or tumors. Tumors are either cancerous or benign. Benign tumors do not penetrate organs in a life-threatening way, nor do their cells travel to other parts of the body. Unfortunately, cancerous or malignant tumors do affect vital organs and their cells can journey to other parts of the body creating secondary tumors.

When cancerous tumors invade organs, they become deadly for basic reasons. If lungs are affected, the body is denied oxygen over time. Kidneys, if cancerous, cannot cleanse the blood in a normal way. A cancerous liver is unable to filter toxins and provide necessary enzymes to maintain the body. Malignant tumors cause organs to shut down and this poisons the body. Cancer by itself creates toxins and this contributes to death. In addition, those with cancer waste away physically as malignant growths feed off their bodies. Death comes about in diverse ways.

Cancer can be massive or pinpoint in size and can resemble cotton candy, golf balls, sponges or other life forms. Textures can be smooth or similar to brain tissue. Tumors can be hard or soft to the touch. Some believe that the size of tumors and whether they are less aggressive or more aggressive (subjective opinions) relate to survivability. This may not be so. It has been suggested that cancer cells reproduce faster than normal cells, but it may be that cancer cells survive or last longer than other cells.

Types. A number of authorities say cancer exists in up to several hundred forms. Cancerous tumors of the breast, prostate, lung, liver, pancreas, stomach, colon, bladder and skin are carcinomas. Standard cancers of the lymph glands are non-Hodgkin's lymphoma and Hodgkin's disease. Leukemia, cancer of the blood, may have its cells originating in the spine. Myeloma cancer is also marrow derived, but occurs as tumors, not malignant blood cells. Sarcomas are the most deadly of all.

Stages. Cancer is categorized by how it has manifested or progressed. Stage 1 (early stage), Stage 2, Stage 3 and Stage 4 (late stage) provide prognoses (data for survivability), and treatments are based on this. Furthermore, Stages 1, 2 and 3 each have ratings of A, B or C. A description of Stage 3B could indicate that cancer is in two areas and has spread to adjacent tissue. Stage 4 (or IV) lacks further classifications for an obvious reason; metastasis (cancer spreading via blood, lymphatics or tissue) would be rampant.

Cancer is rare in children and incidents for cancer increase with age. Most colon cancer occurs in people middle aged and older. Half of all breast cancer develops in women well above age 60. Most men who are 90 or older have prostate cancer, though usually this is not fatal. Perhaps either cancer takes time to develop or the body's immune system declines with aging and this allows for cancer.

Repeatedly, cancer is misdiagnosed. A medical doctor told one man he had cancer but a biopsy by another physician proved the suspicious nodule to be a treatable fungal infection. Cancer cells are usually irregular in shape compared to normal cells, but experts viewing slides often disagree whether cells are cancerous or not. Several million women in America get annual Pap exams (named for a Greek scientist) to detect cancer of the cervix primarily, but tests are often inconclusive. Low PSA (prostate specific antigen) numbers for men don't always mean an absence of prostate cancer, nor do high PSA numbers always prove the presence of cancer. Self-examination is not a method to rely upon, according to many health professionals.

Cancer is not inevitable. Researchers suggest most cancer has an environmental cause; and the strongest association is with food. Less than 10 percent of cancer in humans is attributable to genetics. Even those with genetic markers indicating a high probability for developing cancer often do not get the disease. If cancer is prevalent in someone's immediate family or if gene testing indicates the likelihood of cancer occurring, then for them preventing cancer should be paramount. Even so, preventing cancer needs to be a goal for everyone.

CHAPTER TWO

Treatments for Cancer

Radiation, surgery and chemotherapy are the conventional methods for treating cancer. Hormonal, immunotherapy and gene therapy are methods considered to be alternative. Any of the methods for treating cancer can cause death and some may contribute to the growth of new cancer. Needle or surgical biopsies may spread the disease as well.

With radiation, cancer is bombarded and destroyed, but so too is normal tissue. Surgery involves removal of tumors by cutting with a scalpel. Medical doctors may have a preference for radiation or surgery – believing one works better or that one is their expertise. In most instances, radiation – more precise and able to reach remote areas – is combined with surgery.

Chemotherapy, a collection of extremely toxic chemicals injected into someone's body, is intended to destroy tumors or individual cancerous cells which may have remained after other therapy. Unfortunately, it decimates cells of the immune system and also harms normal cells. Researchers and physicians have attempted to make a science of chemotherapy, but generally it's trial and error. Even though two individuals have the same type of cancer and share body characteristics, what chemotherapy works for one may not work for the other. Treatments may last several months to a year or more, and it's never certain cancer has always been eliminated. Chemotherapy is ineffective for many cancers.

The news media tell of the rich and famous going for treatment to the recognized authority for a specific cancer. Glowing reports allude to a remission or near cure, typically. Then the person dies. Newspaper obituaries show the faces of young and old alike who died from cancer after current medicine could not save them. Surviving cancer with radiation, surgery and chemotherapy (and even for other therapies) is not reassuring.

Nevertheless, many people have lived cancer-free 40 years or more after having received radiation treatment or after having undergone surgery. This occurs more so for those with relatively infrequent cancers which are contained or confined to specific organs or localities. Individuals with blood cancers in the 1950s usually died; most with this cancer today are cured with chemotherapy. The reason for this may be that chemotherapy can "wash over" individual cancer cells in the blood, but tumors may possibly engage a unified defense.

Gene therapy and immunotherapy (inducing the body to fight the disease naturally) offer the best hope for providing a true cure for most cancers. Gene therapy targets cancer cells only, and when perfected will be tailored to each person's genetic distinctiveness.

In previous immunotherapy, interleukin (a hormone of the body) has been used to stimulate the immune system to increase the number of white blood cells to fight cancer. However, Dr. Ron N. Apte, professor of immunology on the faculty for Health Sciences at Ben-Gurion University in Beer-Sheva, Israel, suggests Interleukin-1 (an immune system molecule) may propel growth of cancer by promoting development of blood vessels. Tumors require new blood vessels. A substance that neutralizes Interleukin-1 exists, but it may be counterproductive – Interleukin-1 is part of the immune system's responses or defense.

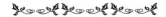

A news wire service reported that a recently developed immunotherapy was able to destroy melanoma tumors entirely in several patients in a small study. White blood cells were removed from cancerous tissue of those treated, and then grown in a laboratory. The new white blood cells were injected back into the individuals. Some who underwent treatment died. A few experienced remission, but this may mean nothing. Yet that almost 30 percent of those treated became cancer-free provides evidence that a cure for cancer can be realized through the immune system. I found this encouraging for obvious reasons, though I was not pleased to learn that chemotherapy was necessary. The report stated that white blood cells extracted from the cancerous tissue recognize cancer as a foreign object in the body, but seemed weakened, unable to do anything about it.

CHAPTER THREE

The Causes of Cancer

Alcohol and tobacco are leading causes of cancer. Remove these factors and incidents of cancer drop dramatically. Why alcohol? When fruits or grains are fermented to make wine, beer or liquor, urethane results as a byproduct. This chemical is tasteless, odorless and extremely carcinogenic (cancer causing). The amount of urethane in any spirit can vary greatly – a single bottle of beer could have a greater amount than a large shot glass of vodka. Drinking heavily increases the possible exposure to urethane, and subsequently, chances for cancer. However, very modest drinking appears to limit incidents of cancer.

Tobacco placed in the mouth causes cancer. Swallowing saliva with tobacco residue contributes to cancer. Cancer from the smoking of cigarettes, cigars and pipes is due to the burning of tobacco – though several hundred toxic additives play a role. Anything which is burned – barbecue, smoked fish, even toast – is carcinogenic. Frying foods produces carcinogens. Cooking almost any food at high temperatures creates carcinogenic acrylamides. Natural sugars in food are responsible for this.

Cancer and industry. Those who work around oil products (gasoline) have higher rates of cancer. Wherever air pollution levels rise, incidents of cancer increase. PCBs found in rivers, lakes, soil, the air and vegetables may cause cancer in animals and humans. Dioxins, from paper products and other sources, and PVCs may cause cancer or may indirectly contribute to it. Close proximity with electrical sources increases risk for cancer. Radiation from past atomic bomb blasts or nuclear accidents may initiate cancer.

Miners who work in asbestos mines often develop a specific cancer caused by asbestos, but many who have spent decades in these mines never develop this cancer or other cancers. Though, a teenager changing the brakes on his car (just once) became exposed to broken asbestos and died within six months from the cancer linked to asbestos.

Cancer and people. Cancer is more prevalent in those who are overweight and physically inactive. Cancer is associated with emotional stress. This could be a reason for the abnormal growth of protein molecules in genes, an expert on cancer said in a television interview. Severe exposure to sunlight or ultraviolet light can cause cancer. Though, not getting several minutes of sunlight during the day may contribute to cancer. Putting pins and needles in the mouth continually causes cancer of the mouth. Frequent use of antacid pills may cause intestinal cancers. Human viruses are linked to certain cancers, and bacteria may cause stomach cancer.

Most cancer of the colon results from polyps or small growths which form there. Only a small percentage of polyps ever become cancerous, but a few individuals develop polyps in a prolific way making cancer almost inevitable for them. This is another way of seeing the problem: if each of 20 individuals has a single polyp in his colon, one would have cancer. Any polyp should be removed as soon as possible as colon cancer takes many lives. Some new methods for discovering polyps may not be safe, but swallowing a camera-in-a-pill may become an easy way to detect polyps.

Cancer and hormones. Anabolic steroids (often used by athletes around the world) can cause liver cancer and brain cancer. Women who are childless have higher incidents of cancer, while women who have numerous children and who breast feed longer have fewer occurrences of cancer. This does not mean that all women who never bear children get cancer. I use this example: 1000 women who have never given birth are compared to 1000 women who have. The women in the survey are similar in every other way. The results may show that over a period of time cancer occurs in 30 more of the women who are childless. Cancer has many other connections with hormones than what has been mentioned.

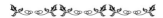

A cousin of a friend died from testicular cancer 40 years ago. He was only 17. Doctors at the time speculated that cancer had been in his body for a lengthy period. Recent research by Gary Schwartz, Ph.D., associate professor of cancer biology at Wake Forest University, indicates testicular cancer results from a male fetus being exposed to Ocharatoxin A or an infant boy exposed to it through breast milk. Ocharatoxin A develops on numerous foods, and can be in cow's milk and pork. Pigs acquire the toxin when they ingest moldy plants or feed; cows obtain it from eating contaminated hay or feed. The toxin may induce lesions in the DNA for cells of the testicles. The mutated cells remain dormant until puberty – the time of hormone development – then become cancerous. However, men with testicular cancer can live for many decades .

Dr. Schwartz believes this cancer could be prevented if pregnant women were given antiinflammatory drugs. Taking vitamins A, C and E could help. **Green tea**, in my opinion, may also be effective in prevention. Obviously, all foods with the potential for having this toxin cannot be avoided, so eating foods and spices which are fresh and uncontaminated is advisable. The problem is the fungus would not be evident to the eye or taste. Aflatoxin, another mold, also causes cancer. Peanuts (especially noted for aflatoxin) are heavily consumed in East Asia and liver cancer is widespread there from this. Rainfall and humidity may be factors in the development of the mold. Peanut oil and additional foods could also have this toxin.

CHAPTER FOUR

The Cold Realities of Cancer

One in four Americans will develop cancer at some time during their life. Other sources say one in three but this seems an exaggeration. Almost half with cancer die within five years. Not much has changed in the last 30 years – humans stricken with cancer today may only persist a year or so longer than those of earlier decades. Statistics for dying do vary with types of cancer, locations or stages. Race, blood type, age and an individual's health are additional factors.

Chemotherapy at times puts cancer in remission. This does not mean cancer is cured but indicates reduction in tumor growth. However, some cells may be more resilient than others, and remission may only mean the elimination of weak cancer cells. If cancer becomes aggressive or supposedly has returned, and chemotherapy is the treatment of choice again, then cancer becomes more difficult to defeat. This is true even when new chemotherapies are introduced. Some have suggested that cancer evolves to become more formidable; others believe the immune system declines from chemotherapy itself. Periods of remission can be months or years, and the time for remissions usually lessen until the inevitable occurs. Moreover, anemia, physical exhaustion and infections regularly result from chemotherapy, and these can be fatal. Radiation therapy is little more than a blow torch, sizzling all tissue it contacts, and most people suffer excruciating pain afterward.

Mammograms. It is not uncommon for women to be diagnosed with breast cancer even after a mammogram (or exam) three months earlier detected nothing – mammograms are judgments, not pure science. If contemplating a mammogram, insist the radiologists be the most competent on staff. Do mammograms save lives? Cancer is detected earlier with mammograms, but there is no irrefutable evidence that lives are saved. I am aware of the very latest studies which say otherwise, but these studies are flawed or compromised – so say other experts. It has been suggested that mammograms contribute to cancer and that a breast exam (possibly thermography) with a health care professional may be a better choice. If abnormal or precancerous cells are discovered (not from a mammogram) in the ducts of a woman's breast, it isn't known if surgery, radiation or chemotherapy would make any difference.

Breast cancer. Total removal of a woman's breast is a radical mastectomy; a partial removal is a lumpectomy. Women with strong genetic evidence for breast cancer occasionally undergo double mastectomies to avoid the disease, but some who do so develop cancer anyway. Currently, 12 states require doctors to tell their patients that mastectomies do not increase the odds for surviving breast cancer.

Several recent studies on new chemotherapies used

on women with breast cancer showed very slight declines in the return of cancer and meaningless increases for surviving five years. Perhaps radiation and chemotherapy permit a few more to become cancer-free or to live longer, but a woman who shouts, "*Yea! Tomorrow is my last chemotherapy*," has no real understanding of breast cancer. Breast cancer is to women what prostate cancer is to men – usually slow developing. Approximately 25 percent of women diagnosed or treated for breast cancer are dead within eight years. However, cancer can return four weeks or 40 years later, and it is almost never ending for women dying. This happens in spite of very latest studies which show that only a very low or modest percentage of breast cancer cells have the ability to form tumors elsewhere in the body.

Prostate cancer. I quote a physician from a television interview, "Surgery for prostate cancer is greatly overdone — it provides considerable revenue for the doctors who perform the operations." Most men, according to him, would be better off to do nothing but be carefully monitored by their doctors. Only if the prostate cancer becomes aggressive should something be done. However, another study said immediate treatment with surgery or radiation would save lives once prostate cancer is first confirmed. It was mentioned there is no test to know if prostate cancer will become aggressive or not. Even so, it is not the case where every man who has immediate treatment for his prostate cancer survives. And surgery and radiation have risks as well.

Health care is about money and cancer treatment is no exception. A Medicare managed HMO plan raised chemotherapy and radiation co-payments from a few dollars to several hundred dollars. Patients who could not afford this went without treatment. Almost 25 percent of Americans are without health insurance or lack meaningful insurance; being diagnosed with cancer with inadequate (or bogus) insurance can have severe consequences. Even those with acceptable health insurance may have claims rejected in certain instances. Furthermore, HMOs may not provide payments for newer, more promising treatment for cancer.

The pharmaceutical companies have created this reality: the drug which blocks a specific hormone from breast tumors costs Canadians less than $30, but in the United States the price can be greater than $200! Be mindful that the American taxpayer may have funded the development of these same drugs. There are those who drive (some go online) to Canada or Mexico for this drug and others, but not all drugs from Mexico are legitimate.

Hospitals or clinics which specialize in treating cancer claim better success for either curing or putting cancer into remission than local treatment centers – the reason being that they have better staffs and utilize the latest treatment. If, in fact, they do have greater success, it may have nothing to do with medicine. As a rule, those who go to special clinics for treatment are prosperous, better educated, open-minded, and more demanding than others. These concepts may ultimately account for the presumed better results.

It has been alleged that some doctors will not refer their patients to other doctors so as not to lose business; and it has been asserted that a few doctors – knowing that treatments for cancer are ineffectual – continue treating their patients just to receive payment. There is also the possibility that these doctors continue with treatment to safeguard themselves from lawsuits. Then again, maybe some of these physicians truly believe it's the best that can be done.

Clinical Trials. Some patients decide to participate in experimental trials after being told they are terminally ill. The outcomes for this are never certain. When undergoing such treatment for cancer, doses of foremost chemotherapies may be increased dramatically, but some methods undertaken may be unprecedented or trailblazing. The National Cancer Institute in Washington, D.C., has information about trials being conducted on every type of cancer. Physicians who administer the trials determine who is eligible. Tel: 800-422-6237. Website: www.nci.nih.gov

A well known hormonal drug may help prevent breast cancer in women, but, the newspaper story added, "maybe not as great as earlier reports indicated." It wasn't mentioned that even though this drug may offer some (actually very little) protection for breast cancer, it may increase risks for other cancer. Newspapers frequently include articles which tell of promising new treatments for cancer, improved methods for testing, or other breakthroughs. "Additional studies must be done" is the usual comment. Such optimism has been perpetuated for more than 50 years, but actual cures seem elusive.

––––––––

The coldest reality for cancer may be that cancer must have some mass or aggregation – lumps which can be felt or spots showing on X-rays – to be diagnosed, but it's usually too late by then. The data from credible sources show that far too many people are not surviving, even when cancer is supposedly "caught" early. Lamentable as it is, incontestable treatments often result only in physicians chasing new tumors and in further anguish and suffering.

CHAPTER FIVE

Food and Cancer

For much of the past one hundred thousand years, the diet for humans would have been bison, mammoth or whatever wild game was available, and periods for hunger were probably unending and extremely irksome. Nuts and root vegetables (discovered by chance) may have been eaten occasionally. And fruit (few even existed) most likely was ignored. I am aware that hunter gatherers eat (or ate) fruit and vegetables, and that chimpanzees, our closest genetic relation, are considered herbivores. (They frequently eat young monkeys.) Yet our ancestors who wandered the plains may have eaten only meat.

Human cultivation of food began shortly after the last ice age ended twelve thousand years ago. The planting of grains, the domestication of wild animals, the advent of dairy production, and the growing of fruits and vegetables should be thought of as recent innovations to the diet for humans. In his books D'Adamo gives a comprehensive explanation of how the four blood types evolved and how food affects each blood type.

Both plant and meat eating animals utilize only a limited amount of the nutrients contained within what they eat – much of the food value passes with body waste. Humans discovered fire and instinctively realized that cooking food benefited them. Their bodies were sustained better and less food had to be obtained. Eating properly cooked food strengthens the immune system and helps prevent cancer. Steaming or cooking for a brief time is favored; many vitamins and nutrients are lost when food is overcooked. In spite of this, raw food may be necessary to provide enzymes. Even when food is cooked at low (perhaps less than 130 degrees Fahrenheit) temperatures, most enzymes are destroyed.

PROCESSED FOODS

Foods which have been dried, flaked, mixed, frozen, canned, boxed, bottled or packaged are prepared foods and should be avoided or limited in the diet. The processing was usually done in the interest of the manufacturer, at times with little regard for the health of the consumer. The Romans, with evidence from two thousand year old skeletons, had perfectly aligned teeth and never any cavities. This was true for senators or slaves. Sugar, white flour and modern processed foods were not in their diet. Wherever sugar, white flour and processed foods (preservatives too) have been introduced, tooth decay, dentures, diabetes, degenerative diseases and incidents of cancer soon followed.

Corn syrup, high fructose corn sugar, inverted sugar, refined cane sugar, caramelized (burned) sucrose, beet sugar and brown sugar are all refined white sugar and should be limited in the diet or avoided. Juices made from concentrates often contain white sugar though the label doesn't always list it. Some families in East Asia keep sugar from their children until the age of 10. They recognize that small children can become addicted to sugar, and denying sugar from them until their brains have developed further appears to lessen the problem. Artificial sweeteners (even fructose or fruit sugar) are very suspect and should be avoided.

Oils. Many commercial oils for cooking have been refined and processed with solvents. Cold pressed, unrefined, additive-free pure oils available at health food stores would be better choices, and consider those oils which comply with D'Adamo's plan. Foods which include hydrogenated or partially hydrogenated oils, fractionalized oil, and palm oil should be avoided as they do not contribute to good health.

Those who consume olive oil have significantly less cancer. Olives are saturated with oil. Solvents or heat are seldom necessary to get the "last drop" which processing companies are intent on getting to increase profits. Extra virgin olive oil is pressed from olives picked from the tree. Other olive oil comes from olives which have tumbled to the ground. These tend to shrivel and solvents or heat may be used. Cold pressed, extra virgin olive oil, dark green in color, and with aromatic taste is preferred. The green sediment in extra virgin olive oil may be antimicrobial; olive oil, unlike other oils, seldom becomes rancid. Olive oil should not be used for frying.

Many health conscious individuals drink milk only if it is raw (not pasteurized or homogenized) and comes from a certified dairy. These dairies must test their cows constantly for disease. Health food stores in a few states are allowed to sell raw milk and dairy products made from raw milk. The 3HO Yogis, a sect of Sikhism whose spiritual leader is Yogi Bhajan, always bring raw milk to near boiling before drinking it. If butter is in the diet, consider organic ghee, a purified butter. There is evidence butter is not unhealthy for many – see D'Adamo's book. Most sources say that margarine should never be consumed. Fertile eggs from cage-free chickens given proper feed (seeds) are also recommended.

Too frequently, breakfast cereals are made from grains which have been bromated, overly milled, drained, roasted and soaked in sugar to provide a long shelf life or to satisfy sugar-addicted children. Many vitamins are lost in the processing; even though a few vitamins are added back, the balance of the grain is never restored. Supplemental iron in cereals is inorganic (unless otherwise stated) and may contribute to cancer. Some cereals and baked goods can cause hyperactivity, mood swings and low energy in children and adults. Such foods should be avoided or limited in the diet.

Luncheon meats, salami, sausages and other preserved meats have been linked to increased risks for cancer. Children who eat numerous hot dogs weekly for considerable periods may increase their chances for developing leukemia. Eat sparingly of pickled foods as these also contain a carcinogen. Though, cabbage, if fermented naturally, can possess nutrients which fight cancer.

Most commercial salt is heated to extreme temperatures enabling anti-caking agents to be driven into it. These table or iodized salts (most prepared foods contain it) have been linked to hypertension and other health problems. Purchase pure sea salt from health food stores, though some sources warn about specific sea salts which may possess toxins. Sea salt – being very salty to the taste – allows many to reduce their intake. Using less salt may lower risks for cancer; however, some people require more salt. There are better sources for iodine than commercial salt.

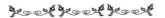

This story is recalled: a surgeon was hunting in a forest and shot a large deer. While dressing the deer, he was amazed at how healthy and red the heart and other internal organs were. As a surgeon, organs of humans he observed during operations were colorless and atrophied. He concluded that people had diseased organs and poor health because the foods they were eating were devitalized.

FISH AND MEATS

Saturated animal fats have a strong connection to cancer. However, the domestic animals of today have little in common with the animals early humans hunted. Wild animals of the prior period grazed on fresh plants and grasses and were constantly roaming. Present animals are grain-fed, have been selectively bred to produce as much meat (fat) as possible, and wander lazily about in pastures or pens. Venison, grass-fed range beef and meat from bison, ostrich and elk contain almost no fat and have been recommended for some in D'Adamo's plan. Pork is not a good choice according to many sources, including D'Adamo.

Hunzas, the mountain people of Central Asia, boil meat in water and discard the liquid, as they believe toxins are in the blood and fat of meat. This somewhat resembles meats which are prepared kosher or Islamic style. In these examples, slaughtered animals have all traces of blood removed by soaking, salting and washing. Many in the world bleed the animals at the time they are butchered. Perhaps these practices reduce incidents of cancer.

It has been suggested that meat contributes to cancer because it remains in contact with the intestines for too long a time during digestion. People who are sedentary should eat less meat and consume more vegetables. Vegetables are alkaline and will offset the acidity (toxicity) of meats.

Fish contain oil which prevents cancer, and eating more fish correct for your blood type is recommended by D'Adamo. Ocean or natural fish is preferred to those farm raised. To know the difference you may have to ask. But wild salmon is beet-red, while salmon from farms is pink. The latter has far less beneficial oil, and may be toxic. Some deep water fish, such as swordfish and similar large species, contain mercury and other heavy metals which can cause severe health problems. Avoid these. The Japanese eat tuna only if it is raw – cooked tuna is considered poisonous. Recent research supports this view.

Question what you eat. Tortillas usually contain lard (animal fat) and one large tortilla could hide a tablespoon of lard within. A popular brand of peanut butter was almost 25 percent lard. The company advertised that its peanut butter was the "richest." It could have added that it was also the most unhealthy. Many are aware that meat is occasionally contaminated with E.coli and listeria, and that cows in Great Britain given feed laced with animal byproducts are responsible for mad-cow disease, for which there is no cure. The news media in America is warning of a potential health problem here – deer are being shot in one state.

GRAINS

Many in the world will eat bread only if it has been baked that day; others insist their bread be baked from whole grain flour which has been stone ground that day. Ezekiel and **manna** bread, both Biblical in origin and kept frozen at health food stores, are made from sprouted grains and have unique enzymes and nutrients. Other breads lack these. Breads which claim to be made from the whole grain or from sprouted grains frequently are not. Read the labels closely and shop at reliable markets. The 3HO Yogis consider most bread to be "dead " and choose to eat freshly baked flat breads. Chinese and Japanese usually avoid bread and consume noodles and other wheat products which have been steamed.

Some should avoid wheat and wheat products totally and limit all other grains extensively. Others do well eating grains. White rice has been steamed previously and vital nutrients have been lost, but this is what most people in the world prefer to eat. Natural basmati rice has not been processed and may be a better choice. Rice makes some hyperactive.

Obtain organically grown whole grains from health food stores and cook these yourself. Grains should be rinsed thoroughly prior to cooking, as washing removes the natural pesticides contained in the husks. Even if not carcinogenic, the toxins would affect the immune system.

Noodles should be rinsed and drained after cooking to remove glutens. These starches can cause intestinal inflammation (celiac) and other maladies. For some, avoiding all grains is the only solution. Be advised! Many processed foods contain disguised glutens. Health food stores sell gluten-free products.

VEGETABLES AND FRUITS

Antioxidants in fruits and vegetables prevent cancer by protecting cells of the body against damage from free radicals (swirling atom-sized irritants). Pigments in the color of fruits and vegetables have healing properties which may also protect against cancer. Most have heard "an apple a day keeps the doctor away" but the follow up states "an onion a day keeps the cancer away." Onions, apples and many other fruits and vegetables contain **quercetin** which is said to be effective in preventing and fighting cancer. Briefly steaming apples will remove harmful oxalates, but will not diminish their healing elements.

Tomatoes in stores are often picked green and sometimes come from Mexico. If from Mexico or overseas, it is uncertain what pesticides or amounts of pesticides have been applied. Eating vine-ripened organic tomatoes or growing your own is recommended. Use natural organic-method bug or fungus repellents if necessary. Tomatoes contain **lycopene** (foods red in color usually indicate lycopene) which may reduce incidents of cancer, including prostate cancer. The skin of tomatoes should be removed as it possesses natural pesticides. (This is true of many fruits and vegetables.) But some should not eat tomatoes at all. Refer to D'Adamo's books.

Green vegetables. Nothing is more healing for the human body than foods green in color, especially leafy green vegetables. Kale and chard are good choices for many blood types – the ubiquitous iceberg lettuce is not good for anyone. Spinach is also recommended for some. It has oxalates like apples and should be cooked briefly – water in the pan should then be poured out. **Parsley** may help prevent cancer – it's recommended for several blood types.

Seaweed, added to soups or vegetable dishes, supplies valuable vitamins and trace minerals, including iodine. A little goes a long way – but I prefer greater quantities. This leafy green vegetable can help control overeating by lessening cravings for carbohydrates, and can also help those with problems of weight gain by regulating the thyroid. Dulce from the waters off the coast of New England (tested for heavy metals and bacterial contamination) is available at health food stores. The seaweed for making sushi is always pressed onto a hot griddle before to kill any microbes or bacteria. Kombu, another variety of seaweed, is a favorite of macrobiotics. Kelp in granular form is the most common seaweed – some use it as a substitute for salt.

Japanese and Chinese value the daikon radish as a healing food. Rutabagas, turnips and parsnips, known in America, are comparable foods to the daikon. These tubers are believed to activate NK cells. However, if ever diagnosed with cancer, it may be better to avoid these foods. Vegetables are a better source for fiber than grains. Frozen (toxins are created) and canned vegetables should be limited or avoided.

Carrots and other root vegetables provide **silica** (a sand-like trace mineral) which benefits the entire body and may help prevent cancer. Silica is excreted through the skin and acts as a stiff brush scouring away unwanted debris. Women in China consume pearls in powder form which is said to make their skin smooth and lustrous – pearls contain silica. Silica is available in liquid form at health food stores, only a few drops are taken.

Vegetarians have considerably less cancer than those who eat meat, though it is a myth that vegetarians have great health and live longer. Mexicans have much less cancer compared to Americans as they eat less meat and consume more vegetables. Japanese and Chinese have fewer cancers overall, which may be partially due to their eating soy products and broccoli, but have higher rates for stomach cancer due to a diet of cured and salty foods. (D'Adamo theorizes the T antigen factor is the reason for this cancer.) Soy does prevent cancer, but recent studies indicate soy products may not be good. If soy is included in the diet, perhaps it should be discontinued for very prolonged periods.

WATER

Food may provide most of the water required by the body, but others say to drink eight glasses of water each day. Dehydration should be avoided, and drinking adequate water whenever thirsty is advised. Drinking too much water when eating may interfere with digestion by diluting gastric juices; macrobiotics suggests limiting water and other liquids at mealtime to quell tendencies for overeating. After waking in the morning, rinse the mouth thoroughly and drink a glass of cool, not cold, water. The Yogis also say just before retiring, urinate, then drink a sufficient amount of water afterward. This keeps the body hydrated while sleeping.

Tap water is not a good choice and well water is often contaminated with pesticides and heavy metals, and may be too mineralized. Water in plastic containers may not be totally free of contaminants, and in fact, carcinogens in the plastic may leach into the water. Some health professionals recommend filtered water. I prefer sparkling mineral water, served at room temperature, with meals, and distilled or spring water at other times. There are those who believe **dis-**

tilled water (the same as rainwater) is best of all. Health food stores sell automatic distillers which will produce one gallon of steamed distilled water per day.

VITAMINS AND SUPPLEMENTS

In America and elsewhere in the world, in much earlier times, most soils would have had **selenium**, **magnesium** and other trace minerals in abundance. Growing crops continually on any soil depletes its trace minerals, as added fertilizers usually do not contain them. Incidents for cancer increase whenever vegetables lack adequate trace minerals. Brewer's yeast is an excellent source for trace minerals, as are organic foods and seaweed.

Coenzyme Q10 (oil and water soluble preferred), **vitamin E, vitamin C, calcium d-glucarate, beta carotene** and B vitamins such a **folic acid** are vitamins and supplements recommended at health food stores, and are believed to lessen incidents of cancer or possibly help in treatment. Other supplements with supposed cancer-fighting abilities are: **silymarin**, a liver cleanser; **whey powder**; **IC3**, derived from broccoli; **L-glutamine**, which boosts NK cell activity; **ellagic acid**, found in grapes and berries; **CLA** (conjugated linoleic acid), occurring naturally in red meats; **pycnogenol**, extracted from grape seeds and pine bark; **fruit pectin powder**; **evening primrose oil**; **genistein**, derived from soy; and **MGN-3®**, extracted from rice husks and shitake mushrooms.

Vitamins should be obtained from reliable health food stores, and megadoses of vitamins and supplements can be harmful. It may be better to get most vitamins (and trace minerals) naturally from fresh organic foods and take only required supplements. Some vitamins may extend lives of cancer patients by many months when included as treatment, which suggests the body can be healed if given what it requires. D'Adamo makes recommendations for vitamins and supplements.

Digestive enzyme combinations, those with **pancreatin**, may help prevent cancer. **Acidophilus** may prevent colon cancer by ridding harmful bacteria in the digestive tract, just as yogurt does. There are acidophilus pills which pass through the stomach and deliver their beneficial flora directly to the intestines and colon. Avoid these pills and others if they contain oils, synthetics, preservatives or other adulterants.

Prescription drugs can remove vitamins and other nutrients from the body, and herbs can interact unfavorably with prescribed drugs. Those who smoke cigarettes and take multivitamins with large amounts of beta carotene increase their risk for developing lung cancer. I have doubts that aspirin prevents colon cancer or other cancers in any meaningful way, but it possibly could.

HERBS

Prehistoric humans relied upon plants for their medicines. Bark from trees, roots, fungi, flowers, weeds, shoots and leaves were steamed or boiled. Even insects, animal parts and fossils were included as remedies. What cured or helped for particular ailments was discovered by observation. Chinese medicine continues this tradition, and many Western medicines are derived from plants. One of the most effective treatments for a particular form of leukemia is extracted from a shrub found in Madagascar. And a new chemotherapy, derived from extremely poisonous American poke root, is now used in treatment for a usually fatal childhood leukemia.

Astragulus, pau d'Arco or Taheebo (the real root and not misrepresentations which are totally ineffective), **ginseng, garlic** (a Chinese herbal doctor said **Aged Liquid Garlic Extract™** is the most effective form), **flaxseed** or **flaxseed oil, omega 3 oil, Sun-Chlorella™** and **spirulina** may help prevent cancer or combat it for some blood types. **Damiana, muira puama** from Brazil, **ashwaganda** and **gotu kola** (both Ayurvedic herbs) are known to increase vitality and virility and are included with treatment for cancer by some authorities. **Cat's claw** (not listed by D'Adamo) from Peru may be an important herbal root for either preventing or curing cancer, and is favored by Europeans. An herbal remedy used to treat prostate cancer was recently taken off the market because it contained prescription drugs.

Many in South Asia consider **turmeric** (botanical name Curcuma longa; **curcumin** is the supplemental extract) the most healing spice of all. It's the main ingredient in curry, and it may combat cancer. I make curry without black pepper but with common curry spices from D'Adamo's plan. Cayenne, also an ingredient in curry, may prevent polyps from forming in the colon, and purportedly strengthens the stomach and improves circulation. Anyone can become accustomed to hot peppers by putting just one drop in food each day for several weeks, then increasing the drops gradually. According to D'Adamo, however, many should avoid hot peppers altogether.

The efficacy of herbs and spices diminishes with age, or if exposed to air, sunlight or heat. Don't leave herbs in a locked car on a hot day even for a few minutes as this will destroy its potency. Purchase only fresh non-irradiated organically grown herbs and spices or grow your own in pots. All herbs and spices should be steamed or heated briefly before consuming. East Asians with vast knowledge of herbs would never swallow a capsule containing a fresh herb. Learn the truth, and don't take herbs mindlessly.

TEA

One in three humans on earth drinks tea daily; even the poorest find a way to include it in their diet. Tea aids digestion, has antibacterial properties and is an antioxidant. There is evidence that drinking black tea and green tea can prevent cancer. Black tea has been roasted and this may lessen its effectiveness in preventing cancer.

To prepare tea, bring pure water to boiling, pour over a tea bag in a pot and wait little more than 10 seconds. Remove the tea bag without squeezing as this increases tannins. One bag will produce three small cups. Pour tea into a thermos and drink later. Asians serve tea in thick glasses, not cups, which allows hot tea to cool quickly. Some suggest only loose tea, not bags, should be used. Distilled water will not produce strong dark tea usually, and this is recommended.

HONEY

Honey, bee pollen, bee propolis and royal jelly are said to aid the immune system. Cancer patients who have undergone radiation treatment or those who have been exposed to radiation may possibly benefit from bee pollen. According to the Yogis, pure organic honey (uncooked and unprocessed and which crystallizes in its container) helps regulate hormones in the body, especially so for women. Keeping hormones in balance may prevent cancer. Honey should not be taken every day and the amount should be less than one fourth of a teaspoon – according to the Yogis. Imported honey contains unfamiliar bacteria (though honey is antibacterial) which may create problems for the digestive tract. Perhaps honey should be stirred in just boiled water for a few seconds before consuming. Still, D'Adamo suggests many should avoid honey and honey-related items completely.

NUTS

Nuts possess zinc, another healing trace mineral noted for preventing or battling cancer. Discolored nuts and seeds are usually rancid and should be discarded. Asians never eat quantities of nuts the way Americans do and eating greater amounts can contribute to constipation or toxicity. Many in Asia consider almonds (only three are to be eaten each day) to be the most beneficial nut of all. Soaking almonds in boiling water for less than 20 seconds – the skin is an irritant for the colon – will allow the skin to be peeled. Walnuts may remove toxins from the body. Yogis consider nuts brain food. D'Adamo lists the nuts suitable for each blood type.

CHAPTER SIX

Lifestyle to Prevent Cancer

 healthy lifestyle and positive outlook can significantly increase the odds for avoiding cancer.

HEALTHY EATING HABITS

Wholesome and unprocessed foods should be eaten every day. A diet of processed foods leads to binge eating and cravings for more processed foods such as fatty, salty and sugary snacks. Avoid foods that are heavy and difficult to digest, and those which have been heated to high (over 250 degrees) temperatures. This includes fried foods, food baked in ovens and even bread and most cereals, including granola. Flat breads are an exception as is manna bread. Manna is baked at very low temperatures for up to 10 hours. The early Hebrews knew this secret but it was lost over time.

For most, eating three modest meals during the day is best. For a few, a light meal in the afternoon settles nerves. Others may benefit from eating a larger meal in the morning. The Yogis suggest eating only one main meal in the afternoon. Waiting at least four hours between meals is usually good advice. Any snacks or light meals should be thoroughly digested before eating a main meal. The Yogis say eat less and you will live longer. Eating less and being active encourages the body to produce heat naturally, and this may also lessen tendencies for overeating. Yogis also say that after eating, the stomach should be one part water, one part food, one part air and one part empty.

Food should be appealing to the eye (harmonious and colorful) and enjoyed. Eat meals calmly, quietly and don't hurry. Europeans eat a small amount of fruit or cheese after a meal to provide them a feeling of being satisfied. One should feel this way after eating. More food could be eaten, but it isn't necessary. A modest bowl of soup after a meal can provide this sensation. For many, soup can shut off cravings for sweets or carbohydrates completely. Place an onion and other vegetables in a mini-blender with some water, then sauté in a pan with a little oil, salt and spices. Eat very slowly. Eat more if necessary. Some may require a small bowl of soup with every meal. Adding small amounts of meat, beans or grains may be warranted.

Cook healthily. Macrobiotics recommends cooking food in Corning Ware®, Pyrex® or heavily sealed pots. Toxins are created when certain foods are cooked in copper, aluminum or stainless steel pans. Non-stick pans shouldn't be used. Consider using ceramic spoons or chopsticks which do not produce the metallic taste stainless steel spoons and forks do. If canned foods are necessary, choose cans which are lined on the inside, as unlined cans allow toxic metals from welded seams to leach into foods. Eating foods kept in the refrigerator for days is not healthy.

Place foods far in the back of the refrigerator where it is coldest, and store leftovers in well sealed glass containers. Microwaving meat, dairy products and even vegetables is not recommended. However, the best health practice is to eat exceedingly fresh foods cooked only for that meal – leftovers are not saved.

A rule for fat in meats: take the skin off chicken before cooking it. Cut off all fat from meat or skim it during cooking. Remove solidified fat from meats cooled in the refrigerator. To acquire extra lean meats (grass-fed beef) or exotic game, seek out specialty markets or health food stores which feature these. People drive hundreds of miles every week to obtain these items. It has been suggested that when eating meat, green leafy vegetables, onions, garlic and ginger be included.

Digestion. Having good digestion may prevent cancer. Sipping a little warm tea before eating calms and prepares the stomach for digestion. Don't make a habit of eating food which is cold. People in their early 40s secrete less digestive acids and this can contribute to health problems if lifestyle or diet is not altered. Coffee may promote good digestion for some but many should avoid coffee completely. D'Adamo provides a thorough explanation as to who benefits and who doesn't. Herbal teas such as peppermint and rose hips aid digestion for some, but only in a limited way. Herbal teas should be drunk warm, not hot. A very small glass of red wine or sparkling mineral water with a meal may help.

The Yogis suggest eating an orange 45 minutes before eating. I prefer five to 10 drops of gentian (a bitter) in water prior to a meal. This is an excellent digestive aid for my blood type. On occasion I take a few drops of gentian after eating. I discovered DGL (deglycyrrhizinated licorice) years ago. It's also a recommended digestive aid for Type O.

Intestinal gas and bad breath are telltale signs of undigested food and improper food combining. Eating milk products with grains is not healthy. Dairy products do not combine well with meats and fruit may not complement grains. It may be better for some to eat fruits or drink fruit juices between meals. But having a strong digestive system or taking digestive supplements may allow some to eat almost anything.

Organic foods (even teas) are recommended. To my knowledge, there isn't an absolute guarantee that organic vegetables have not been grown on soil previously contaminated with toxic waste or poisonous fertilizers. Soils for growing organic foods do have requirements, however. Organic foods should look and taste great.

WE LIVE IN A DANGEROUS WORLD

Rubber gloves and breathing masks offer some protection when handling cleaning solutions and other chemicals. Avoid secondhand smoke from cigarettes and stale air in houses or offices. Check for radon or carbon monoxide where you live and store household chemicals in the garage. If living in a mobile home or trailer, be aware of the possible danger from urea or formaldehyde. Keep the house free of germs. Question everything you breathe or contact. Plates or cups could contain lead – test for this. Even chocolate contains some lead.

A TV report recently told of multiple childhood leukemia cases showing up in a "cluster" area of a town adjacent to an air force base. The leukemia may be the result of jet fuel being burned by planes flying overhead. Children came down with a form of leukemia which requires powerful chemotherapy which is often unsuccessful. The people who live there say they are worried but are determined to stay. They would be better off to move.

Nine people working in an large office building contracted cancer over a short period of time. Statistics suggest one case of cancer would be normal. Power sources in the building would be primary suspects. Continued close contact with televisions, radios, computers, cell phones (an ear plug may offer some protection) and other electrical devices can increase incidents for health problems and cancer. Computerized Axial Tomography (CAT) scans may also contribute to cancer according to several sources. Gold jewelry contaminated with uranium, unbeknownst to the wearer, can cause chronic illness and possibly cancer.

PERSONAL CARE FOR THE BODY

Practice good dental hygiene; bad gums and teeth lead to additional health problems. Rinse with warm salty water and not with commercial mouthwashes. Root canals may increase risks for cancer. Metal fillings may also contribute to cancer. Consider plastic composites for teeth, but make certain they are free of heavy metals and aluminum. The front teeth can be used to scrape mucous from the tongue, or use a tongue cleaner. This mucous should never be swallowed.

The "monkey glands" located behind the throat should be cleansed every morning and other times if necessary by clearing the throat or coughing. Fatty meats or heavy meals especially eaten late in the evening contribute to the accumulation of phlegm here. Hot coffee or tea should not be used to wash this mucous down. Swallowing these toxins (bacterial meningitis can be present) would only increase stress for the body. Even if the tonsils have been removed, these glands remain.

Never ignore nature's call. Delaying may contribute to constipation as the body is constantly extracting water from fecal matter for the small intestines. One or two bowel movements daily is normal for many, but this depends on amounts, types of food and individuals. Being constipated, straining at the toilet or having incomplete evacuations does not make for good health. Primordial humans relieved themselves by squatting on the ground and Turkish toilets (holes in the floor) are common in the world. Constipation is seldom a problem with this method. Constipation is omnipresent in the West with sit down toilets. Training the body with squatting exercises during the early morning and at other times could help. Encourage the body to urinate after eating. Urine should not remain in the bladder any longer than necessary and flushing it regularly may prevent bladder cancer. Keeping the body alkaline will also assist.

Dependency upon chemical laxatives or even herbal remedies should be avoided. Eating greater amounts of green leafy vegetables, especially steamed spinach, and fruit (prunes, stewed dried figs, mangoes) and limiting grains should produce regularity. Drinking fresh vegetable juices would be beneficial. Continued use of psyllium is not recommended, nor is added bran in the diet. The occasional use of a small teaspoon of ground flax seeds with a meal can help. The Yogis of 3HO say that stools which float in toilet bowls indicate nutrients are being assimilated. If stools sink, vital nutrients are passing through the body and are not being utilized.

The Romans of the thousand year Roman Empire bathed daily for several hours; at least this was true for the elite or privileged class. Roman baths consisted of three pools, one of ice-cold water, one of hot water and one lukewarm. Some would have entered the lukewarm pool first, then dunked themselves into the hot one. A final plunge would have been in the cold pool. Bathing in this manner relieved stress, aided digestion and eliminated toxins from the liver and kidneys. Modern saunas and hot tubs do the same. This may not be something to do too often, however.

Wear comfortable non-restricting clothing; fashion should never come before good health. Women with tight-fitting bras may increase their risk for breast cancer. The wearing of suspenders should be considered by some men. Sandals may prevent more than foot pain. Good posture is essential; keep the back straight and head level when sitting or walking.

EXERCISE

Exercise reduces incidents of cancer, perhaps more so than any other preventative method. Our early ancestors walked great distances, ran, crawled, climbed, squatted, threw objects, lifted, stretched, twisted, leaned, pushed and carried large packs over hills and through valleys daily, all the while breathing fresh air. It is quite likely they experienced little cancer. The body is meant to be exercised thoroughly each day to where it sweats profusely – according to the Yogis. Vigorous exercise helps maintain a strong immune system, and keeps food moving through the digestive system making bowel movements more regular and thorough.

Joining a health club isn't necessary; exercises can be done at home. Olympic style medicine balls may be of benefit. Power Systems®, Inc. has medicine balls of every weight and type. Fit balls and other exercise devices are also available. Contact the company at: P.O. Box 31709, Knoxville, TN 37930. Tel: 800-321-6975.

SLEEP

Sleep is important for good health. Go to bed early. Limit television or reading before retiring. An autosuggestion that one will sleep soundly and awaken refreshed can help. Some deep breathing routines and simple stretching exercises just before bed are beneficial. When sleeping, do not become too warm or too cold. Wear all cotton long nightclothes. Sleep on a very firm bed. Placing a hard cushion between the legs while sleeping is a remedy for lower back pain. The 3HO Yogis say one should fall asleep the moment the head touches the pillow. Also, according to the Yogis, the head and feet of the body should be positioned east to west to maintain the correct electromagnetic field.

Being stressed or eating heavy meals in the evening can produce poor sleep – undigested food in the digestive tract at night may contribute to cancer. Caffeine in coffee, tea or chocolate can interfere with sleep. Alcohol and salty foods can dehydrate the body and interrupt sleep. Don't rely on sleeping pills, but occasional use of herbal remedies may help. Many claim to benefit from drops of melatonin. If insomnia remains after a change in diet and lifestyle, seek medical attention; insomnia is a serious health problem. Working at night disrupts the biological clock and may cause hormones to fluctuate. If night work is necessary, sleep in a totally dark room during the day or cover the eyes, and make certain sleep is deep and adequate. Proper exercise will help as well.

The Yogis say that upon waking one should get out of bed after taking several deep breaths and doing a few stretching exercises. Sleeping late in the morning and taking long naps are not advised. A brief nodding off in a chair or curling up on a couch for just a few moments after a meal may be of benefit. I prefer to stretch out on the floor on my stomach for five minutes.

How much sleep is needed? Six hours of sleep may be adequate for some, while others may require eight hours. With better health practices, sleep could be lessened and one could feel better.

THE SKIN

A very attractive woman almost 60 years of age was interviewed on TV. She learned from her mother never to go outdoors without a hat and always to cover her hands, arms and legs. She had no sun damage to skin or hair whatsoever and appeared to be 30 years younger than her biological age. This woman probably will never have skin cancer. Childhood sunburns can come back to haunt one decades later with skin cancer.

Any suspicious lesion should not be ignored. If one has numerous moles, be aware of the dangers. Some moles should be removed as a preventive measure. Teens, pregnant women, and those who are stressed can experience skin eruptions, the result of hormone imbalances and toxicity. A healthy lifestyle and correct diet should prevent most of these problems. Tanning at salons is not a good idea.

The skin breathes and absorbs whatever is placed on it. Bug repellents or other aerosols should not be applied to the skin. Wear long clothing and spray this if necessary. Consider wearing cotton clothing which can be washed – some believe synthetic fabrics should not contact the skin. Clothes dry cleaned with solvents most definitely should be avoided. Cosmetics which contain mineral oil should not be applied to the skin as the oil is inorganic and will clog pores. Natural oils encourage the growth of new skin. Use a few drops of cold pressed olive oil or almond oil. I prefer walnut oil with a fragrant essential oil. Other unadulterated oils may do as well to moisten skin when necessary. Lotions, shampoos or soaps containing DEA are to be avoided. The use of natural mineral underarm deodorants should be considered. Avoid any with aluminum.

Physicians often prescribe skin creams to treat skin cancers which do not usually metastasize. There is promise of skin creams which may reverse DNA damage to the skin and which may prevent breast cancer, or be included with treatment. I have used SkinAnswer to remove brown or reddish-brown age spots from hands and arms. Health food stores special ordered it for me. A daily application for three or four weeks was necessary to get positive results. Follow the instructions if using it.

Remove calluses from the soles of the feet or elsewhere with pumice stones. Yogis say nerves connect the solar plexus with the feet and rough skin on the soles can interrupt the flow of energy and lead to serious illnesses. Walking barefoot on stones or rough concrete is invigorating, but walking barefoot on grass sprayed with weed killer is not advisable.

HEALTH PROBLEMS

Recent studies and health practitioners suggest many over-the-counter drugs are ineffective, toxic and should not be used. Articles in newspapers often say prescription medicines are over prescribed and have far too many dangerous side effects. Several hundred thousand individuals are believed to die each year from taking medications. A few health publications –

written by physicians – believe that some prescription drugs could be replaced with natural remedies. Do further research and do not cease taking any prescribed medications without consulting your qualified medical practitioner. If possible, take the path which allows natural foods and a wholesome lifestyle with a minimum use of drugs to provide good health.

Herbal remedies for any ailment must be taken with caution. Herbs can have side effects like drugs. Ma huang – containing ephedra – can cause death, and kava kava, the most potent herb known according to Chinese herbalists, can cause permanent liver damage if used continually. A woman discovered that certain herbal supplements prevent her hair loss; what had been provided by dermatologists did not help. Seek proper advice. Herbal remedies can be helpful but may not solve all problems. Herbalists frequently suggest that herbs be discontinued for periods of time. Also, herbs, unlike other medicines, can take days, weeks or months to work. Fruit, if taken at the same time, may lessen the effectiveness of some herbs.

STRESS

A task one person accomplishes in a relaxed way and finds satisfying is regarded by another as stressful. Some cope with stress by facing their fears or acclimating themselves to challenges. Many find it best to avoid stressful situations entirely. D'Adamo's plan may lessen stress and his recommended supplements and natural tranquilizers could also help. (Blood Type AB should heed this advice.) Exercising and maintaining a healthy lifestyle would complement this, making stress manageable for most.

Listening to music which mimics the human heartbeat helps alleviate stress. The tabla, a small drum beaten by hand and frequent in music from India, provides this beat. Having a dog or other pet and taking long walks can combat stress. A good laugh everyday – not at the expense of others – helps relieve stress. A brief crying spell can rid tension for some. Spending quiet evenings is also recommended. Breathe fully during the day and allow stress to flow from the body on the exhale. Those who breathe in a shallow way develop health problems in the stomach and bowel areas. Gossiping, emotional upheavals and anger are to be avoided if stress is to be kept out of someone's life.

Be cognizant of tension which can hide in the shoulders, ribs or neck. Massage these places with your fingers. Seek massage therapy if necessary. Forceful adjustments by a knowledgeable chiropractor can be helpful. Alternative Asian medicines recognize that blockages of energy in the body can cause stress and illness. Many claim to have benefited from hands-on therapy of acupressure, Reiki, Shiatzu, Reflexology and Rolfing.

Hypnotherapy has been used by many to quit smoking and to cease other bad habits which contribute to stress. Bulletin boards at health food stores list those who offer this. Aromatherapy, the science of fragrant smells, may help relax muscles and calm the mind. A morning shower with an Auyervedic soap or applying essential herbal oils (appropriate for your blood type) can provide this.

People who do not develop cancer:

1) Avoid tobacco.
2) Don't drink or drink moderately of alcohol.
3) Enjoy their work and see their work benefiting others.
4) Keep stress to a minimum.
5) Go on trips for relaxation and return refreshed and rejuvenated.
6) Don't dwell on the past and don't harbor resentments.
7) Keep from anger.
8) Have a good laugh during the day.
9) Have an interest in current (hopefully accurate) health information.
10) Seldom eat fried foods, processed foods or refrigerated food.
11) Eat fresh steamed leafy green vegetables daily, usually organically grown.
12) Eat modestly.
13) Have and maintain good digestion.
14) Get adequate pure salt.
15) Eat seafood several times a week.
16) Exercise vigorously daily and rest afterward.
17) Practice good health routines.
18) Get perfect sleep and rise early, ready to face the world.
19) Eat a light dinner early in the evening.
20) Practice a one day fast during the week.
21) Limit fat intake, especially fat from bad sources.
22) Limit or avoid sugar.
23) Take precautions with chemicals.
24) Breathe correctly.
25) Enjoy being outdoors briefly, while protecting their skin from direct sun.

26) Do not live in polluted cities.
27) Are active, yet know how to relax.
28) Remain positive about life no matter what happens.

PEOPLE WHO DEVELOP CANCER:

1) Are angry.
2) Hate their jobs.
3) Have poor relations with others.
4) Blame the world for their problems.
5) Sleep poorly and are tired during the day.
6) Eat devitalized foods.
7) Seldom exercise.
8) Eat burned foods and fatty foods.
9) Eat late at night and go to bed with undigested food in their system.
10) Binge drink or drink continuously.
11) Go on trips and return more tired than when they left.
12) Snack before and after meals, especially eating quantities of fatty, sugary, salty and packaged foods and drinks.
13) Have indigestion.
14) Have constipation and/or diarrhea.
15) Smoke cigarettes, pipes or chew tobacco.
16) Breathe erratically.
17) Take no precautions with solvents, bug sprays or other cancer causing chemicals.
18) Are depressed.
19) Have poor health habits.
20) Are overweight and out of shape and go from one diet to another.
21) Seldom get fresh, appropriate green leafy vegetables.

22) Are not optimistic about their future.

23) Are not positive about life.

24) Are aging before their time.

25) Are haunted by past traumatic events.

26) Continuously seek over-the-counter medications.

27) Get little natural sunlight during the day.

28) Are sedentary.

29) Are emotionally distressed.

30) Breathe stale air in closed environments.

31) Have a toxic body.

CHAPTER SEVEN

Diagnosed with Cancer

M any with cancer rush to undergo the ac cepted treatments, demanding to get through their plight as soon as possible. With cancer the situation is perilous, requiring serious deliberation. Three consultations with very qualified health professionals are usually advised before deciding on treatment. It has been recommended that the doctor who made the diagnosis should not be the one who provides treatment. Be heedful that surgeons tend to recommend surgery, while radiologists are inclined toward radiation therapy.

Know the consequences of treatments beforehand. A woman underwent surgery and received chemotherapy for breast cancer. The cancer returned 12 years later. She then learned chemotherapy often permanently damages the lining of the lungs, and consequently, certain alternative therapies were not available to her. A local newsman developed cancer and his doctors suggested an aggressive treatment program. The one with cancer believed this approach was reasonable. However, treatments of radiation and surgery severely damaged his stomach. He was free of cancer, but lived in great discomfort and died 10 years later from the effects of the aggressive treatment. Other doctors may have chosen a more cautious path, but it is impossible to say if this would have saved his life.

Support groups. Most support groups are stringently overseen by hospitals or organizations which have direct ties to established medical facilities. Alternative health associations see a conflict of interest with this, and tell of pressuring by these health facilities on those patients who are doing research and contemplating other treatment. The ones who "sell" conventional treatment often receive a hefty commission. Independent support groups do exist. Any support group can be helpful provided you are not networking with people who are just as ill-informed as you about cancer.

Perhaps the meek will inherit the world one day, but they will not survive cancer. If you have cancer, you cannot turn your life over to others and expect them to fix it. Be fully aware of what treatment entails; and know the authority you are giving to any physician. Catastrophes can and do happen. Anyone can ask specific questions about chemotherapies and seek opinions from other professionals. Chemotherapy, perhaps few dollars for the actual chemicals, costs tens of thousands of dollars when delivered as treatment. Someone's costs or profits should not be influencing treatment you require. Know that just as chemotherapies differ, types of radiation vary.

If you are contemplating chemotherapy, a medical laboratory in Long Beach, Calif., will test recently obtained biopsies with appropriate chemotherapies.

The idea is that if cancer cannot be destroyed in test tubes, then particular chemicals injected into someone's body will not kill cancer there. Better to have tissue samples as the "guinea pig," not you. Still, there are risks with biopsies.

Some are told to refer to the cancer in their body as "my cancer." Therapists say the reality of the disease must be accepted. I consider cancer to be nothing but dumb, worthless cells. I don't need to know the facts about dying from cancer. I choose to know about those who are alive and well, about those who survived even when their doctors said nothing more could be done.

Having cancer means that you should not continue with what you have been doing. If you are a smoker or drinker, this must cease for you to have a better chance of surviving. Yo-yo diets, excuses, poor sleep, and a hectic lifestyle must end. Clinging to bad habits may make any therapy or treatment program unsuccessful. A man in his thirties, 50 pounds overweight and worried about surviving cancer, was interviewed on television. He was in his kitchen baking rolls made with white flour, white sugar and heavy oils. These very foods may have contributed to his getting cancer. I am pessimistic about his chances.

Cancer does not care that you are a good person or that you are a mother with two children who need you. Even the cancer industry has no sympathy for those with cancer. Putting up a "heroic battle against cancer" or "dashing for a cure" counts for nothing. Those diagnosed with cancer should have cool determination, stop seeing themselves as victims, and use logic and knowledge in choosing therapy. One physician said it is the patient alone who ultimately makes the final decision regarding treatment.

CHAPTER EIGHT

Alternative Therapies

History of medicine. Bloodletting was the unquestioned and standard treatment pre scribed by recognized health practitioners (some even Harvard trained) for millennia. This incomprehensible methodology helped kill George Washington! Surgeons performing operations in America for centuries gave no thought to cleaning their instruments or washing their hands. Surprisingly, not all of their patients died. When germs and viruses – even the deadliest – were first observed under microscopes, the established medical world dismissed them saying, "Something this small couldn't possibly be harmful."

At the turn of the 20th century, a researcher in Germany discovered the four blood types but 10 years passed before a medical researcher in New York City came upon his study, and then gave an explanation why some died from transfusions and some got better. Lives were then saved. Another medical researcher toured the South in the early 1900s and determined that a poor diet (foods lacking B vitamins) caused pelagra, a painful flare-up of the skin which habitually ravaged the faces of thousands of men, women and children. A decade elapsed before his work was acknowledged. Better diets were then suggested and pelagra was ended.

In 1992, parents of a small boy were told by doctors that nothing could be done for their son who was diagnosed with the rare progressive brain disease Adrenoleukodystrophy (ALD). He would soon be crippled and die. The mother and father, after doing intensive research, created a remedy which they named Lorenzo's oil – mostly olive oil and rape seed oil. Their doctors scoffed at the notion. The boy eventually became disabled, but he survived. Researchers verified 10 years later that the therapy of oil indeed works. Those with ALD who receive treatment with the oil before symptoms appear go on to live normal lives.

The future for cancer. Someday, surgery, radiation and chemotherapy – the primary conventional methods for treating cancer – will be wholly abandoned. Cancer will be ended in an effortless way. Even now, researchers and physicians who treat leukemia anticipate that a pill may soon replace dangerous bone marrow transplants. Many cancers may prove to be preventable with vaccines or genetic engineering for the immune system.

Alternatives. Most of the remedies discussed can be prescribed by medical doctors. Doctors with knowledge of alternative (or complementary) remedies can be found in the Resources section. Moreover, read the books which are mentioned for complete and accurate facts. A few therapies listed require physicians to include chemotherapy in treatment, even though doctors might prefer not to do so. The following are either health practices or alternative therapies.

ISCADOR

Iscador, derived from mistletoe, has been a permissible remedy for cancer by doctors in Germany for years. It was banned in the United States, until actress Suzanne Sommers and others campaigned successfully to make it legal. Mistletoe is poisonous if eaten.

WHEAT GRASS

As a health aid, wheat grass juice powder and barley grass juice powder are available in glass jars at health food stores. To produce fresh wheat grass juice, organic wheat berries are spread evenly onto wet organic potting soil. The seeds are then sprinkled with added moist soil. Several wood boxes 30 inches x 18 inches in size, and filled two to three inches deep with soil, are adequate for the task. When watered adequately and correctly and kept in the shade, the grass grows to five or six inches in height within a week, just as lawns do.

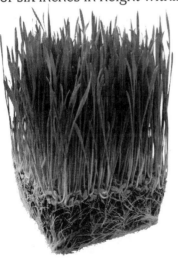

Each box will yield two clippings. One method is to put the cut grass in a blender with some water, and then strain afterward; however, health food stores offer automatic and hand operated wheat grass juicers. Those with grass allergies should avoid these items. There are physicians in America who include wheat grass juice in treatment for cancer.

Eydie Mae (Hunsberger) Loeffler, along with her

husband Chris Loeffler, wrote *How I Conquered Cancer Naturally*. Up until 1975, Eydie Mae Loeffler had survived very deadly breast cancer for almost three years with wheat grass juice and a diet of raw foods. She learned this health routine at Ann Wigmore's natural healing facility in Boston. Here, wheat grass was ground to produce the juice. The fresh juice was also used in retentive (held in) enemas. For this, a warm water enema was completed first. An enema bag fitted with a tube or catheter, and only partially filled with wheat grass juice, was inserted. The juice was released into the upper bowel, seemingly with natural pressure. Retained for a brief period, it was then expelled. Mrs. Loeffler provides daily usage information and tells her method for growing wheat grass. Her book was republished in 1992. Apparently, she was still living.

In her original book Eydie Mae Loeffler spoke of a doctor who said wheat grass juice contains abscisic acid known to inhibit growth of tumors in studies. The Fort Worth Public Library (science section) said abscisic acid regulates and influences plant growth and promotes dormancy in leaves. It affects plant transpiration, stress responses, germination of seeds, and embryonic genesis.

MUSHROOMS

Many in East Asia believe the **shitake, reishi** and **maitake mushroom** can prevent or cure cancer. Only these exotic mushrooms possess plant steroids known for developing muscles and endurance. The steroids may increase the activity of NK cells to eliminate cancer. East Asians regularly eat a bowl of soup made with several of these mushrooms as a preventative. **Kombucha** (a fermented mushroom drink) is featured at health food stores and may fight cancer. Some consider the supplement MGN-3 to be a mushroom product and a remedy for cancer.

Russians, likely from an obscure region, make a 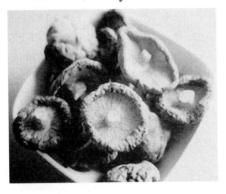 tea from a fungus that grows on the bark of the white birch tree. The fungus contains a glycoside that is either digitoxin or a glycoside much like it, and it may either prevent or help cure cancer. Digitalis, the ground leaf of **foxglove** *(Digitalis purpurea)* whose active substance is digitoxin, was used as a heart medication years ago. Recent research and tests indicate digitoxin (not the synthetic form digoxin which is completely ineffective) should be considered as treatment for cancer. Digitalis in a proper dose is harmless. This is a partial excerpt from an article titled *The Anti-Cancer Effect of Digitalis* by Wayne Martin, and was published in *Cancer Victors Journal,* Vol. 23 No.3, Winter/Spring 2001. Martin is a research scientist and often writes about alternative cancer treatment. For further information contact: Wayne Martin, 25 Orchard Dr., Fairhope, AL 36532

SHARK CARTILAGE

East Asians also believe shark fin soup will prevent or cure cancer. Several hundred million sharks give their fins for this assertion each year. Shark cartilage may prohibit the growing of blood vessels to tumors, and may also stimulate cells of the immune system.

While I was at a health food store, a woman came in and shared her story. Doctors informed her that surgery, radiation and chemotherapy for her cancer had failed and she was terminal. Someone suggested shark cartilage as a possible remedy. She is 78 years of age and has survived eight years. A bottle of shark cartilage capsules lasts her two

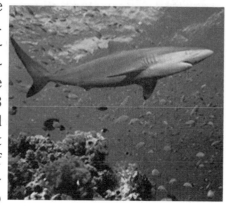

weeks. It's not known if this woman changed her diet or included additional therapies or remedies. She was cheerful and appreciated living immensely.

On another occasion, a health food store owner told me of a woman with a cancerous tumor the size of a golf ball in her chest. She took shark cartilage powder. The tumor shrank considerably and no other malignancies appeared. Doctors advised her to do nothing but continue with checkups. A year later she insisted the tumor be removed. After surgery, the tumor was found to have been encased in mucous and no longer capable of growing.

Kay Bevan, with her husband John, wrote *Learning To Love My Cancer*. Kay has survived terminal ovarian cancer more than 10 years with shark cartilage. She went to Mexico for treatment once. Retentive enemas of shark cartilage were used earlier. She now takes shark cartilage powder on a completely empty stomach 45 minutes to an hour before eating. Stomach acids, they believe, lessen the effectiveness of the cartilage. At one time the amount of shark cartilage taken was increased significantly. Chemotherapy may have damaged her digestive system making enzyme supplements crucial for her now. I was told Kay is Blood Type A. The book is published by Charhill Voice, LLC, P.O. Box 344, Sonoita, AZ 85637-0344.

John Bevan is familiar with a man with pancreatic cancer who was given six weeks to live, but is fine now, having taken shark cartilage. He said thin people seem to do better with shark cartilage, and that the cartilage doesn't work well for women with ovarian cancer – perhaps helping only one third. Shark cartilage may be effective for prostate cancer. There is no evidence to corroborate any of his beliefs, and the Bevans never prescribe treatment.

BeneFin™ manufactures the microprocessed shark cartilage preferred by the Bevans. *Sharks Don't Get Cancer* by Dr. I. William Lane, tells of studies done on shark cartilage and includes possible procedures. The cartilage may act synergistically with other treatment, and now exists in an injectable form. Bovine cartilage, according to other studies, may be more effective. Articles written by Dr. John F. Prudden on bovine cartilage can be found on the Internet. See Alternative Health Watch. Bovine cartilage did not help Kay Bevan at all, according to John Bevan. Shark liver oil may also have anti-cancer properties.

MACROBIOTICS

The macrobiotic diet consists of 60 percent cooked whole grains such as organic brown rice or organic wheat, five percent to 10 percent soups, 20 percent steamed vegetables, 10 percent or less of beans or legumes. Seaweed or sea vegetables, seasonings and condiments are included. Little oil is used in cooking. Sesame and corn oil work well for sautéing. Macrobiotics does not allow dairy products, eggs, or beef. Fish can be eaten occasionally. Fruit is limited and bananas are excluded. Barley syrup or rice syrup as sweeteners may be used infrequently in very small amounts. No sugar, honey or molasses is permitted. Umeboshi plums are considered extremely healing. Vegetables not peeled are scrubbed diligently with firm brushes.

Macrobiotics encourages those on the plan to do internal cleansing every so often. Almost no oil, sweeteners or fruit are taken for a brief period. (This can be very challenging.) Macrobiotics contends that juice from specific leafy green vegetables is superior to that of wheat grass juice or wheat grass juice powder as a health aid. The juice of leafy green vegetables should be boiled briefly in a ceramic pot and allowed to cool before consuming. According to macrobiotics, nutrients are not destroyed.

The following macrobiotic books offer information about cancer prevention and treatment: *The Macrobiotic Way* by Michio Kushi. *Cancer Prevention Diet* by Michio Kushi. This includes recipes and practical advice for relieving 25 types of cancer. *Macrobiotic Approach to Cancer* by Michio Kushi. 12 personal accounts of recovery from cancer. *Nature's Cancer Fighting Foods* by Verne Varona. *Macrobiotic Miracle* by Virginia Brown. Recovery, through macrobiotics, from melanoma. *When Hope Never Dies* by Marlene McKenna. 10 years cancer-free from terminal melanoma with macrobiotics. *Physician Heal Thyself* by Dr. H. Faulkner. A doctor survives terminal cancer. *Confessions of a Kamikaze Cowboy* by Dirk Benedict. Turning from meat eater to macrobiotic vegetarian saves him from prostate cancer. *Recovery from Cancer* by E. Nussbaum. A personal story of triumph over uterine cancer. *My Beautiful Life* by

Mileneka Dobic. She survived Stage 4 ovarian cancer with macrobiotics.

Cooking lessons and counseling are provided at the Kushi Institute. Cancer patients go there periodically. For a catalog of macrobiotic products, books or information contact the Kushi Institute. Tel: 800-645-8744. The George Ohsawa Macrobiotic Foundation publishes a magazine and also provides books on cancer prevention and treatment. The foundation, like the Kushi Institute, has organizations around the world to advise on macrobiotics. Dr. Kieichi Morishita's book *The Hidden Truth of Cancer* is available from the Ohsawa Foundation. Morishita ardently believes that cancer cells can be transformed back to being normal cells with macrobiotics. Tel: 800-232-2372.

ESSIAC

Apparently originating with Native Americans, Essiac became a treatment for cancer in Canada, but was eventually banned there. I have read testimonials from those who claim to have been cured of cancer with the herbal formula tea. *The Essiac Report* by Richard Thomas has the details. Essiac tea is available at health food stores as a liquid. Preparing the tea from fresh herbs (steaming it too) could possibly make it more efficacious. In most instances this remedy would be in disagreement with D'Adamo.

THE MOERMAN DIET

Dr. Cornelius Moerman, in Holland 70 years ago, created this diet to treat his cancer patients. It resembles the macrobiotic approach with whole grains and fresh vegetables, but dairy products are allowed. Vegetable juices are taken between meals. Innumerable people claim to have been cured of cancer after following

Moerman's regimen. Read *Dr. Moerman's Anti-Cancer Diet* by Ruth Jochems.

LAETRILE

Apricot seeds can cure cancer? There are stories or rumors that say this is possible. Apricot seeds, apple seeds, sesame seeds, beans and legumes contain what is known as Laetrile (Vitamin B_{17}). Wheat grass or barley grass would have Laetrile in abundance. Evidently, drying wheat grass juice at low temperatures to produce powder preserves its Laetrile. Bona fide sprouted grain breads would have considerable amounts of Laetrile. Barley syrup and organic brown rice syrup would be sources for Laetrile. The rice syrup (processed with a fungus) would also be a source of beneficial enzymes for a few blood types. The microscopic amount of cyanide in Laetrile may be responsible for the destruction of cancer cells, and may also spur metabolic activity.

Injections of Laetrile are given by alternative health practitioners in treatment. Several cancer survivors listed in The International Association of Cancer Victors and Friends, Inc. (Resources section) say Laetrile injections were included in their therapy. An example was provided by a son:

Frank Willey, an engineer, retired at age 60 in 1978 and was soon diagnosed with adenocarcinoma of the colon. Doc A recommended surgery and this was scheduled with Doc B at a hospital. Frank and Doc A met with Doc B and discovered the latter was inebriated or on drugs. Doc C removed the tumor and 18 inches of colon, a sigmoid colostomy. Chemotherapy was refused. The cancer returned and spread in 1979. Doc D said Frank had one to three months to live with or without surgery and chemotherapy. Frank heard on the radio about clinics in Mexico practicing alternative medicines. He traveled there and met Dr. Ernesto Contreras of Centro Medico del Mar and received metabolic therapy. No pain was experienced. Faith was encouraged. A colostomy irrigation was given each morning. No alcohol was allowed. No smoking. No coffee. Fresh fruits and vegetables were on the daily menu. An exercise routine was required. There were no dairy products, salt, meat or fried foods. But fish was allowed and chicken with its skin removed. **Amygdalin** (extracted from bitter almond seeds and leaves) injections were given three times per week. The tumor was gone. Six years later markers indicated a recurrence. Treatments were then begun weekly. Frank Willey remained in remission for the remainder of his life. He passed away at age 82 of congestive heart failure. Mr. Willey may have published a book titled *An Engineer Beats Cancer.*

IP6

"Discover the new antioxidant with the power to prevent and fight cancer!" proclaims AbulKalam M. Shamsuddin, M.D., Ph.D., in his book *IP6: Nature's Revolutionary Cancer-Fighter.* IP6®, derived from the B vitamin inositol, increases the activity of NK cells. Rice, corn, wheat and soybeans are sources of inositol. According to Dr. Shamsuddin, IP6, alone or combined with inositol, can kill cancer cells, shrink tumors, and boost the body's immune system. Shamsuddin markets IP6 at health food stores.

Entelev, Cancell or Cantron
Medical Research Products offers Cantron and G-H3 (the original formula of Professor Ana Aslan, M.D.). For literature Tel: 305-628-0981, 800-443-3030.

GERSON DIET (NON-PROFIT ORGANIZATION)

The Gerson Institute provides cancer therapy at its facility in Bonita, Calif. Every type of cancer, from melanoma, cervical, breast, lung, prostate, non-Hodgkin's lymphoma, to bone cancer, has been reversed, even for those at "death's door," with the Gerson Diet™. Founder Dr. Max Gerson began this therapy more than 60 years ago and believed that a malfunctioning liver and pancreas (organs which break down and assimilate food) are the cause of cancer. Treatments consist of drinking vegetable juices, eating organic meals, and taking vitamins, minerals and herbal extractions daily. Salt must be limited as this affects vital potassium. Coffee enemas are frequent and retentive chlorophyll enemas may be recommended. Injections are given at the facility. *The Gerson Healing Newsletter* is published monthly. Books, tapes and lists of physicians with knowledge of the diet are included. Those who intend following the plan at home may find this helpful. The Gerson Diet plan suggests individuals not work for two years if possible. For a brochure Tel: 619-685-5353.

Marilyn Barnes Bloom worked for the Gerson Institute for many years and offers counseling by telephone or with personal contact. Her advice is to read Gerson's book *A Cancer Therapy* first. Marilyn had Stage 4 melanoma 22 years ago and has remained on the Gerson plan since. Request fees. Tel: 925-682-3982.

THE TIJUANA CONNECTION

For years, Americans have crossed the border to seek treatment for cancer at dozens of clinics in Tijuana, B.C., Mexico. If a newly developed treatment in the United States or overseas shows promise, but the Food and Drug Administration insists on a decade-long study before granting its approval, then such treatment may show up in Tijuana. Some facilities there are staffed by qualified medical practitioners, many American or trained in the United States; while other clinics are questionable and will administer treatments, suitable or not. Most who go there are in poor health from the effects of radiation, surgery, chemotherapy and advanced stages of cancer. Yet some treated there say they were cured when medical doctors "back home" said nothing more could be done. The Resources section lists those with firsthand experience at the clinics.

Peggy Pousson has been conducting tours to Tijuana from San Diego since 1978. She knows the clinics, doctors, nurses, the doctors' wives and even the custodians and kitchen staffs. Tel: 619-475-3834. Website: www.healthtours.com.

Vitamins, sometimes as an intravenous injection, are included in treatment. Shark cartilage in large doses is given. **Hydrazine sulfate** is mentioned – it may block sources of energy for cancer. **Germanium,** Laetrile, **DMSO** are provided. Vegetable juices, along with potassium salts, are frequent. **Hyperthermia**, when blood is extracted, treated, then injected back into the body, is another treatment. An additional form of hyperthermia treatment will be discussed later. Coffee enemas are oftentimes required.

PURGE THE PARASITE, CURE THE CANCER

Hulda Regehr Clark, Ph.D, N.D., in her book *The Cure For All Cancers,* says cancer is caused by parasites and microbes. Dr. Clark suggests bacteria, carcinogens (propyl alcohol in the liver) and a weakened immune system contribute or interact with parasites allowing them to enter cells in the host body where they pass through several stages of development. The parasites originate with undercooked meats, vegetables, dried or fresh fruits and milk. Even water is suspect, according to Clark. Pets can be responsible for microbes. Dogs have heartworms and other parasites, and these have stages of development. Viruses and microbes, found within parasites, also have stages of development.

Clark believes an herbal concoction of **Black Walnut Hull tincture, wormwood and cloves** will eliminate parasites at all their stages and end cancer. Clark is adamant about using the word "cure" and not treatment. She adds that once parasites have been removed, the weak and toxic body must be restored to good health rapidly, or parasites return and cancer results again.

The book cover states that Clark received her doctoral degree in physiology in 1958 from the University of Minnesota and that she has been a research scientist in biophysics and cell physiology since that time. Another book by her is *The Cure For All Advanced Cancers*. Her books are available at health food stores. She maintains a clinic in Tijuana.

An anecdotal letter was passed along to me: a family dog was diagnosed with colon cancer. Funds were limited, so treatment was ruled out. Dr. Clark's book was recommended by a neighbor and the dog was given Black Walnut Hull tincture with wormwood and parsley – *not cloves*. The vet insisted the dog would live but a few months. But the bleeding stopped and the tumor disappeared. The dog regained its energy and was soon back to playing. Everyone at the vet's office is surprised when the big dog is brought in for its annual shots. The dog is given the tincture combination periodically in its food as a preventative. The letter is on file.

POLY-MVA

Dr. Stephen Sinatra, a physician with an impressive background listed in his brochure, declares: "The biggest breakthrough in the war against cancer...Pull the trigger and kill any cancer cells in your body...Poly-MVA™ is even better than antioxidants for cancer PREVENTION." And "For full instructions on how to take Poly-MVA and where to get it, see my *Cancer Prevention & Healing* report, which is free with a subscription to my newsletter. The faster you put this advice into action, the lower your risk of cancer will be." Poly-MVA is, from reading his initial brochure, "a natural substance – a unique combination of the element palladium and **alpha lipoic acid** – and has absolutely no side effects, unlike radiation, chemotherapy or surgical removal." Three testimonials from those who used Poly-MVA to become cancer-free are provided. Tel: 800-861-5970 for information about the *Sinatra Healing Report.*

GENE THERAPY

Dr. Stanislaw Burzynski created a cancer therapy whereby **antineoplastons**, originally taken from blood and urine and now synthesized, normalize cell development in a genetic way. The following is from his literature which is available upon request: "Antineoplastons are non-toxic, naturally-occurring peptides, amino acid derivatives and certain organic acids that fight cancer with few if any side effects. Rather than poisoning cells like traditional chemotherapy, antineoplastons act as biochemical microswitches, turning off the genes that cause cancer (oncogenes), activating the genes that fight cancer (tumor suppressor genes)." "Antineoplastons ...we find profusely in the blood and urine of healthy people, but see only in scant amounts in the blood and urine of persons with cancer." Numerous publications tell of individuals with almost always fatal cancers who have been cured with this therapy. For information contact: Burzynski Research Institute, 9432 Old Katy Road. #200, Houston, TX 77055. Tel: 713-335-5697. Website: www.cancermed.com. Ancient herbal healers from India discovered that drinking one's own urine cured certain illnesses, and this remedy is widely practiced there today. Urine contains hormones and is antibacterial.

—————

A woman, 70 years of age, diagnosed with inoperable lung cancer was given chemotherapy. This was discontinued after one or two treatments when she had severe reactions. Doctors told her to go home and enjoy her grandchildren – in other words, *die.* Her sons went on the Internet and discovered a medical doctor who utilizes **P53 Gene Therapy** in treatment. They contacted him and she was given this therapy. The tumors in her lungs stopped growing; she has survived five years.

JUICE FASTING

Dr. Rudolph Breuss, in his book *The Breuss Cancer Cure,* believes **a vegetable juice diet *only* for 42 days will cure cancer.** Breuss' theory states cancer cells cannot exist more than 42 days without complete protein which only meat, fish, eggs and dairy products provide. Breuss maintains that over forty thousand of his patients in Austria and Germany were cured of cancer with his plan. A crushing-style juice extractor is required – juice from centrifugal juicers is diminished. Weights of the vegetables are exact, and tea formulas are explicit and intended for specific cancers. Consult his book for details.

Anne Fråhm is a survivor (surgery, chemotherapy and bone marrow transplants all failed) of breast cancer. Read her book *A Cancer Battle Plan* with David J. Fråhm. She directs Health Quarterly Ministry in Colorado Springs, Colo. For information about eight-day juice fasting retreats contact the organization. Tel: 719-593-8694.

FLAXSEED OIL

Johanna Budwig, Ph.D., in her book *Flaxseed Oil As A True Aid Against Arthritis, Heart Infarction, Cancer, and Other Diseases,* gives a precise account of how fats play a role in maintaining good health and, if not in correct balance, lead to cancer and other degenerative diseases. Dr. Budwig has specific diets and provides numerous testimonials. Read her book for details. Flaxseed oil contains linoleic and linolenic acids, the substances believed to provide the health benefits. Flaxseed oil is not used when cooking, only added afterward. Health food stores carry both oil and seeds.

THE POWER OF THE MIND

Years ago, a man from my hometown was terminally ill with colon cancer. This was told to me by a good friend who attended Catholic school with one of his sons. Doctors advised the father to get his affairs in order, go home and accept his fate. Instead, he consulted with a doctor in Dallas who included **visualization** in therapy. To the amazement of all, the cancer went into remission and disappeared. The family of this man became very distressed as he left their church and joined a faith-based fundamentalist organization. Members of this group had participated in the visualization study. It is my understanding that the individual with cancer lived long into old age.

Many have heard or read similar accounts. Doctors often say cancer was misdiagnosed and had never existed. But others are convinced cancer did exist and that something did occur for the cancer to vanish. Divine intervention? Or can the mind heal the body? Certainly what someone thinks can bring about illness, but could the mind wish cancer away?

In 1984, Greg Anderson was told he would die in one month from widespread lung cancer. Anderson had been an executive for Dr. Robert Schuler, the TV minister and pastor of the Crystal Cathedral (Garden Grove, Calif.), and knew the value of **positive thinking** well. Anderson is alive today and heads The Cancer Recovery Foundation of America. The non-profit organization has an extensive list of books and programs which may benefit one with cancer. *The Cancer Conqueror* was written by Greg Anderson. To contact the organization write:

P.O. Box 238,
Hershey, PA 17033.
Tel: 800-238-6479.
Website: www.CancerRecovery.org

Other approaches to positive thinking could be of benefit. Dr. Wayne Dyer offers his version of *A Course in Miracles*. Stephen Covey and Norman Vincent Peale are additional authors to consider. Libraries are a source for books on realizing one's inner potential. Hypnotherapy, self-hypnosis, biofeedback and auto-suggestion are other possibilities for either acquiring motivation or controlling pain.

Curanderos, Mexican folk doctors, use hallucinogenic mushrooms to treat those who come to them with physical or emotional ailments. These natural healers guide the ones with health problems through their illness. Once the cause of the affliction is known (quite predictably an evil spirit) then healing begins. The **power of faith** should never be underestimated. I have no knowledge of anyone being cured of cancer by a curandero.

THE SECRET IS OXYGEN

Deep sea divers rely on hyperbaric oxygen chambers. People recovering from operations benefit from breathing pure oxygen from canisters. Clinics in Europe, Cuba and Tijuana claim great success in treating cancer with oxygen. I recently learned of a clinic in the Czech Republic which also utilizes oxygen therapy in treatment. The oxygen used is medical ozone – not atmospheric. A small amount of blood is withdrawn, ozone is added, then the blood is injected back into the body. Ozone may increase the effectiveness of antioxidants and enzymes if these are taken at the same time.

Several individuals in books listed in the Resources section say they were cured of cancer with intravenous injections of various forms of oxygen therapy. Food grade hydrogen peroxide and magnesium oxide are mentioned. Handling either can be extremely hazardous. Hydrogen peroxide is available in three percent and 30 percent strength.

VACCINES

An afternoon newsbreak reported that a newly developed vaccine has proved 100 percent effective in preventing cervical cancer. A form of human papillomavirus (HPV) causes an infection of the cervix, and almost all cervical cancer results from the long-term effects of HPV. The vaccine prevents HPV. Within five years, very young female children will be given the vaccine, and presumably, they will never experience cervical cancer during their lifetime. One medical doctor described this as "an amazing event."

At a North Texas medical facility, vaccine therapy (immunotherapy) is currently being enacted on those with folicular non-Hodgkin's lymphoma. Cancer tissue is removed, treated and then returned to the person's body. There are no side effects and progress has been reported. The facility is optimistic this approach may be effective against other cancers in the future. A similar vaccine study, also in Texas, is being conducted on prostate cancer.

Clinics in Tijuana use vaccines in treating cancer. Cancer cells are extracted from the patient and a vaccine is developed from this within several weeks. The immune system is said to be reeducated to recognize cancer. Protective elements of cancer are removed allowing cells of the immune system to penetrate and destroy the cancer.

After reading Dr. D'Adamo's book, I immediately received the **vaccine which prevents pneumonia.** The Livingston Foundation Medical Center (Resources section) includes vaccines in its therapy; other facilities or physicians do as well.

ENZYME THERAPY

Many practitioners of alternative medicine include enzyme therapy (both injections and supplements) in their treatment of cancer. Aging, overeating, consuming wrong foods and being sedentary can lessen the production of natural enzymes and health problems can result. Some who take enzyme combinations rave about the benefits. Injections may be more effective for those with cancer.

Margé B. wrote that almost six years earlier she was diagnosed with ovarian cancer (Stage 3C). After surgery, she was given Carboplatin™ (a chemotherapy known for unbearable side effects – a librarian read this to me) and taxol (derived from a plant). Her physicians bluntly informed her that she would live 14-18 months. The treatments were continued but she consulted with a medical doctor who was also an N.D. He treated her with bimonthly B_{12} and folic acid shots, plus additional injection therapy. Dark Field Live Cell Analysis was included. Enzyme supplements, Vitamin A, Vitamin C, Coenzyme Q10, zinc and other B vitamins were added to her diet. He encouraged her to rest, relax, sun herself, exercise, adopt a better diet, give up sugar, and set her life in a positive manner. This is what she did, evidently. Currently, she sees the naturopath twice a year. She said two doctors told her to tap her thymus gland a couple of times each day to stimulate her immune system. The thymus lies below the base of the neck. An animal thymus used as food is called sweetbread, and D'Adamo considers sweetbread from cattle highly beneficial for Blood Type O.

HYPERTHERMIA

Cancer cells are vulnerable to heat. With hyperthermia, radio waves of temperatures of 107 degrees to 113 degrees are aimed precisely at cancerous tumors. The following is from Dr. Haim I. Bicher's Valley Cancer Institute's brochure: "In normal tissues, blood vessels open up (dilate) when heat is applied, dissipating the heat and cooling down the cell environment. Unlike healthy cells, a tumor is a tightly packed group of cells and circulation is restricted and sluggish. When heat is applied to a tumor, vital nutrients and oxygen are cut off from the tumor cells. This results in a collapse of the tumor's vascular system and destruction of cancer cells. It is more effective with radiation and chemotherapy and is mostly pain free. New techniques and improved equipment have been developed in the last few years. The therapy is noninvasive and treatments last one hour and are applied daily for up to six weeks usually." For information, contact

Valley Cancer Institute
P.O. Box 66549
12099 W. Washington Blvd. #304
Los Angeles, CA 90066
Tel: 310-398-0013

MARIJUANA

Marijuana, either as treatment or to lessen pain from cancer or treatment, is legal in a few states. Marijuana contains two active ingredients; one encourages relaxation, while the other produces hallucinations. It isn't clear if either makes a difference regarding treatment. Several with inoperable brain cancer are purported to have survived long-term with the use of marijuana. Dr. David Williams, in his February 2002 health newsletter *Alternatives*, mentions a study which showed those with adrenal cancer (almost always fatal in two to three years) survived decades by smoking marijuana daily. The amounts mentioned were considerable. Contact him about his newsletter. Tel: 800-219-8591.

CHINESE REMEDIES

Chinese remedies of **herbs, moxibustion, T'ai Chi, Chi-kung (Qi Gong),** acupressure and other methods may either cure or put cancer into remission. Studies in the West have confirmed that many Chinese herbal and health remedies are effective in treating cancer. Four individuals interviewed on television – all had refused surgery, radiation and chemotherapy – said they were cancer-free, 10 years later, after relying on Chinese methods.

At a health food store I was told of a woman in Dallas – a vegan or strict vegetarian – who when diagnosed with breast cancer, delayed surgery and consulted with an N.D. This doctor inserted a needle – possibly **acupuncture** – into her breast where it remained bandaged for some time. The procedure may have been repeated. She returned to the doctors who made the original diagnosis, and they were unable to detect the mass discovered before. I am still attempting to verify this story. A Chinese herbalist said to me that for good health water in the body must flow unimpeded. Illness comes about when water is blocked. Acupuncture is intended to remove blockages, so that water and energy become free-flowing again. The psychological aspect for this should not be disregarded.

GERMANIUM

Germanium – said to be a powerful antioxidant and immune builder – is found in organic broccoli, seaweed, garlic and several other vegetables. Ginseng has been mentioned as a good source. Health food stores market **GE-132®** (available in liquid form and as capsules) which contains pure organic germanium. A young woman working at a health food store told me she personally assists a customer who has been taking germanium for four years for a cancerous tumor of the pituitary. The tumor remains but continues to lessen in size. Germanium (a trace metal, not a trace mineral) can be toxic if taken in extremely large doses.

Julia H., in 1978, developed health problems and evidence of precancerous cells when tested. Then, in 1986, doctors told her she was terminal with pancreatic cancer and had but weeks to live. Germanium was extremely important for her initially. She later included it with carrot juice, wheat grass juice powder, a grapes diet and numerous supplements. Julia once made a trip to Mexico for treatment. Her Christian faith was important too. She is 73 years old, successfully operates a one-woman accounting-tax preparation service in North Carolina, and is in excellent health. This was told to me in a letter, though I spoke with her briefly once. The germanium originally taken by her may have been extracted from coal, and would be considered inorganic. The Food and Drug Administration banned germanium at one time, but Julia petitioned Senator Jesse Helms and it was kept legal and available.

CHAPTER NINE

Healing Cancer Naturally

In a realistic but make-believe study, 20 individuals with an exceptionally deadly cancer are tracked or followed. All receive surgery, radiation and chemotherapy, but this proves unproductive and treatments are stopped; doctors say none will live for long. Less than 18 months later, only three remain. Another six months pass, two now survive. Five years after the study was initiated, just one is alive. Then, 25 years later, this now elderly individual dies from natural causes while asleep in bed. I naively asked my dermatologist during a checkup: Why is it someone always survives cancer even when treatments fail? He knew this was true. Shaking his head, he replied, "It's a mystery. No one knows."

Shark cartilage, diets of organic food, fasting with juices, mind power, Laetrile, exotic mushrooms, bark from a tree in the Amazon forest, Chinese medicines and numerous herbal concoctions have cured someone with cancer somewhere at sometime. There is ample evidence for this. Although, in limited clinical studies (few alternative methods have ever been tested), no individual has ever been shown to have been cured, though some did have their time for surviving extended. Several alternative researchers claim the trials were conducted improperly and unfairly. It should be remembered that conventional medicine is not a fail-safe treatment for cancer either.

There must be a scientific explanation – a common thread – which reveals what has taken place in those who are cured with alternative methods or who survive when treatments do no good. In the fictional study of 20 individuals with cancer, I envision the 19 who died enduring physical pain, fear, exhaustion, anger, loss of appetite, deteriorating health, depression and poor sleep. They worried about the future for their families. They never had peace of mind. Any hope or spirit faded, and they withered away.

What about the lone survivor? The survivor may have accepted the verdict of dying with a shrug. Perhaps this individual became withdrawn, but not depressed. Maybe the television and radio were turned off. Newspapers or books were no longer read. The telephone was disconnected and most contact with humans was avoided. The survivor ate sparsely and instinctively of the right foods. Evenings were spent relaxing in a chair with no distractions. The individual went to bed early and awoke long before the sun rose. Quiet walks and watching birds in the trees were normal activities. Emotional upheavals were unknown. Maybe faith was relied upon. The years drifted by; the survivor waited for death from cancer but it never came.

Where others agonized, the survivor chose detachment and **serenity**. Having a tranquil state of mind may be a significant factor for those cured through natural methods or who survive when treatments fail. Cancer is associated with hormones pulsing erratically, either too much or too little. When the lone survivor "gave up" and retreated within himself, perhaps his body was returned to balance. Normal cells may have ceased responding to cancer, and at the same time, NK cells and other protecting cells of the immune system were energized to fight the disease. The effect of going into an emotional neutral possibly overwhelmed the cancer or kept it at bay. In his book Dr. Max Gerson stated "a normal body has additional reserves to suppress and destroy malignant cells."

Last week, I spoke with friends in Australia. He said everything was fine. But his wife confided he had leukemia. Everyone is amazed at how well he is doing emotionally and physically. I later recalled he is a Seventh Day Adventist. He does not work on Saturday and the entire day is spent contemplating. For the remainder of the week, stress of any kind is avoided. He may have developed cancer of the blood from holding the power line of a jackhammer between his legs for 12 years. His faith, avoiding stress and relaxing may be helping to keep him alive today.

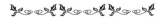

There are other possible explanations for surviving with alternative methods. Shark cartilage, wheat grass juice, Laetrile, macrobiotics and vegetable juice bring abundant nutrients to the body, one of which is calcium in its purest form. It could be that a weakened body readily absorbs this pure calcium and is calmed in a unique way. Infants given breast milk are sedated by calcium and soon fall asleep. Sleep releases growth hormones which repair and build the body and maintain the immune system. Alternative remedies may do something similar. Calcium may calm the body; hormones which assist in healing may then be released, and the body goes about the task of fighting the disease. Plus, cancer is associated with inflammation. Calcium, or other nutrients, may be anti-inflammatory and this may help rid cancer.

Alternative therapies may empower normal cells to seal off nutrients, enzymes or oxygen necessary for cancer. In this way, natural therapies may act as a less destructive chemotherapy. Kay Bevan, after taking shark cartilage, pleaded with a brain surgeon to remove a tumor which developed in her brain. He derided her use of alternative remedies and gave her no chance of surviving with or without the operation. Nevertheless, after her relentless pestering, he agreed to perform the surgery. In the midst of the procedure, he discovered that the tumor had calcified – he had to chisel it out. It was later determined that the tumor was benign – statistically only a remote possibility. It would be conjecture to say the tumor was strangled or starved by the shark cartilage.

Most vegetarians believe eating meat causes or contributes to cancer. However, not all who adopt a vegetarian diet avoid cancer. And some who survived with natural remedies did not become vegetarian – Margaret Fenzel is an example. Regardless, most alternative methods remove meat from the diet which allows the digestive system to rest (meat is difficult to break down) and encourages the body to mend or fight cancer.

Hormones in meat may fuel tumor growth. Not eating meat may be similar to hormonal drugs or therapies which block estrogen from breast cancers for women and deny testosterone from prostate cancers for men. In addition, amino acids in meat may sustain cancer. Most vegetables and fruits lack the amino acids of protein, but avocados, brewer's yeast, nuts and a few other foods do. It may be wise to avoid these foods if cancer exists. However, Julia H. ate brewer's yeast and meat when recovering.

Seeds. Laetrile, flaxseed, IP6 and organic brown rice (central to macrobiotics) are derived from seeds or are seeds. The elements in seeds most certainly boost the immune system to fight cancer. Maybe elements in seeds produce antineoplastons in the blood which Dr. Burzynski recognizes as a cure for cancer. Or possibly these natural remedies influence or balance hormones and this provides a cure.

Supposedly, cancer has a negative charge as opposed to normal cells which have a positive electromagnetic charge. Most people who develop cancer consume devitalized foods and stress robs the body of what few vitamins are in the diet. Many alternative remedies replenish the body with vitamins and nutrients quickly, and this may influence the electromagnetic field making cancerous cells positive. It's more likely that relaxation accounts for balancing the body's energy field, but nutrients certainly assist.

In earlier chapters on foods, lifestyles and therapies, the concept of balance is everywhere. Foods which are adulterated or processed are unbalanced and contribute to cancer. Pure foods prevent cancer and are helpful in curing cancer. A balanced lifestyle prevents cancer; balancing hormones may cure cancer. Those individuals who turned to alternative methods (or survived when conventional treatments did not work) bolstered their body's metabolism and reversed a biological disorder, allowing them to survive cancer.

A NON-TOXIC BODY

A person's alkaline/acid balance can be tested and those with cancer have exceedingly high levels for acidity. Many alternative authorities believe the body must be returned to being more alkaline if the battle with cancer is to be won. I was subjected to a lifetime of intense stress and body toxicity. Grains are acid forming for my blood type (possibly more so for non-secretors) and eliminating these from my diet removed the cause of stress and toxicity almost completely. My body is more alkaline now than when decades ago I ran three miles each day and included an hour of yoga as well.

Reducing food intake moderately, eating foods appropriate for your blood type, and exercising correctly can return the body to being more alkaline. Juice fasting can also do this. With juice fasting, organs of the body are allowed to rest. Stored toxins resulting from overeating or from incomplete digestion are either purged or burned by the body. Enemas are necessary with fasting, otherwise toxins from body waste are reabsorbed.

When the body is in proper balance, body odor and clothes which appear to be "sour" after worn for a day cease. Underarm deodorants may be unnecessary. The skin feels amazingly clean. There is no "morning breath." The mind is clear and one is energized in a spontaneous (non-caffeine) way. This is evidence for a non-toxic alkaline body and one which may offer the best possibility for fighting cancer. Those who survived cancer with macrobiotics, the Gerson Diet, the Moerman plan or similar diets may have made their bodies less toxic. Most who elected to follow these diets probably were not Type O, or if they were, likely had strong digestive systems. This kept their bodies more alkaline.

"Don't You Want to Live?"

I have been asked what I would do if I were diagnosed with cancer. Some are noticeably shocked when I say that I have no confidence in surgery, radiation or chemotherapy and would refuse them. They respond with, *"Don't you want to live?"* I tell them that they should get the facts about cancer and read the statistics for surviving with conventional treatment. Surgery is very reasonable for removing a melanoma from the skin – but doing this may not solve the problem. On the other hand, conventional treatment for cancer of the colon, pancreas, liver, brain and for melanoma cancer discovered within the body is something else altogether. The odds are extremely unfavorable in most of these situations. Death is almost mandated.

For me, I would consider the Breuss Cancer Cure (drinking fresh organic vegetable juices) at the beginning. Only, I would not consume vegetable juices or herbs which are on D'Adamo's avoid list for Blood Type O. I could persevere for 42 days if this was necessary with juice from spinach and other appropriate vegetables. In years past, I fasted with vegetable juice for up to 10 days at a time. But, if digestion was poor, I would consider heating the juice briefly. Steaming the juice would allow for quick assimilation.

Why not Breuss altogether? Breuss spoke about patients who did not do well in treatment; he believed this was their fault in not following his diet. Most of Breuss' patients would have been Blood Type A – this blood type experiences more cancer. The diet he proposes is suitable for Type A, but is much less agreeable for Type O. Most of his patients who dropped out were probably Type O. Breuss paid no attention to blood types and was inflexible with therapy.

A crushing-style (not masticating) vegetable juicer had been recommended before. Juicing vegetables in this manner may produce enzymes similar to the way garlic must be crushed in order to activate its enzymes. Breuss adds that if sediment in the juice is not removed with a fine strainer, then cancer may not be overcome. Sediment could hinder complete digestion and allow for a hangover of nutrients (natural sugars) which would allow cancer to flourish. Carrot juice is known to "scrub" the system. IP6, Laetrile, germanium or other supplements which are reported to fight cancer, if taken with carrot juice, may be removed and not utilized. Juice from other vegetables may not do this.

Enemas would be included with the juice fasting regimen. Whether it is necessary for so many to be done (some clinics require four to a dozen each day) is debatable. I am familiar with a yoga concept in which a very tiny amount of cayenne (beneficial for Type O) is added to water for enemas. Only those who have consumed considerable amounts of hot peppers daily for years could do this. Retentive enemas of chlorophyll would be of interest. Most liquid chlorophyll is derived from alfalfa which is an irritant and avoid for me. Parsley juice could be an option, but there are other choices.

A newspaper article about the use of a caffeine derivative to successfully treat skin cancer in a study made me reevaluate coffee enemas. Coffee, a roasted product, would be carcinogenic and I dismissed it immediately. However, Dr. Max Gerson in *A Cancer Therapy* said that such enemas were essential to clear the liver, not stimulate peristalsis. When drinking coffee, caffeine may be negated in the stomach just as ingested shark cartilage may be offset by stomach acids. Enemas of coffee would deliver unaltered caffeine directly to the colon, and it is caffeine which may help surmount cancer. The sparking of metabolism (or flushing of the liver) by caffeine could also contribute to the defeat of cancer. Gerson and other clinics which administered coffee enemas in therapy must have noticed that those patients who received it were the ones who survived cancer more often. Gerson explicitly stated that 30 drops of caffeine should be added to its recommended castor oil enema solution. Dr. D'Adamo's research suggests that coffee can be beneficial for Type A. Again, Type A has more incidents of cancer, and this would help explain why it was preferred by clinics.

Colonic irrigations. Colonics are extremely useful for cleansing the intestinal tract. I would consider this therapy. I know two people who were scheduled for operations to remove most of their colons due to chronic bowel inflammation or Crohn's disease. Colonic irrigations and changes in diet reversed their conditions completely, saving them from unnecessary surgeries and permanent disabilities. Most facilities which offer this are listed in the *Yellow Pages*. However, the Gerson Diet warns against high colonics – potassium is affected. Health food stores offer numerous supplements or programs for cleansing the colon. I'm familiar with most.

Other fasting. I once did a water fast for 24 days. I had intended doing it for 28 days but was unable to continue. Lengthy water fasts would not be considered again, as they can cause irreversible kidney damage, and even dying is possible. Nor would I do a fresh grape juice fast for 30 days, though I know those who have.

Cancer must be put into remission, but perhaps this should be done gradually. Tumors which are dead or dying are extremely noxious for the body. If not disposed of or reabsorbed in a calculated way, they could be lethal. I might stay with a juice diet for several weeks, then pause and consider other possibilities. I alternate with numerous preventive remedies and supplements throughout the year now. Although D'Adamo doesn't say, Black Walnut Hull must be either a beneficial or neutral for my blood type. Under no circumstances would I return to a grain-based diet. I would not I drink wheat grass juice nor I would not take shark cartilage, but other blood types could possibly benefit from these.

At some time the body would require protein to maintain itself. I might boil meats I'm familiar with in water and pour out the liquids – B vitamins would then be necessary. From reading promotional material, I learned that grain-fed cattle have almost no CLA, while grass-fed cattle possess vast amounts. CLA keeps fat from accumulating in the muscles and elsewhere. This may help balance hormones, and could explain why some believe it combats cancer. This may not benefit blood types other than Type O.

Kay and John Bevan's book reveals the ordeal of their learning about alternative methods, trying them and then discovering they didn't help. John told me they were lucky that time didn't run out before they located what did work for her. Others who survived were equally tenacious and overcame obstacles with perseverance and resolve. I would do the same.

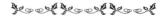

Diets, supplements and remedies listed in the Chapter for Alternative Therapies, or mentioned elsewhere in the book, can be matched against the spices, vegetables, herbs, supplements, fruits and grains which are categorized in D'Adamo's plan. For example, flaxseed oil is beneficial for both Blood Type O and Type A, and is included in Dr. Budwig's recommended remedy. Milk thistle is a beneficial for Blood Type A. Silymarin is an herbal supplement derived from milk thistle and is used to treat prostate cancer. Perhaps, those of Type A would benefit. However, this is only speculation on my part. It is possible that silymarin or milk thistle could worsen the conditions for cancer. Seek professional advice.

If a food or herb is recommended by an herbalist or nutritionist, but is to be avoided according to D'Adamo, I wouldn't use it. However, enzymes and particular supplements are not restricted by considerations of blood type. IC3 should be acceptable as a possible preventative or cancer-fighter because it is derived from broccoli, a beneficial food for all blood types. Again, I'm merely speculating. Don't rely on this.

Yogi Bhajan said, "Why use a sledgehammer when a tap would do?" Resorting to extremes could be disastrous. This applies to vitamins, supplements, herbs, antioxidants, over-the-counter and prescribed medicines, foods and all other remedies. Any of these on their own or in combination could be harmful if cancer is present. The November 2002 edition of *Life Extension* referred to a study in *Cancer Research, 2002, Vol 62, Is 9, pp 2474-2477,* which indicates genistein negates the intended effects of tamoxifen.

Kay Bevan consulted with both MDs and NDs and was tested systematically to know her condition. Others who survived cancer did the same. This certainly would be an advantage, otherwise instincts and observation would have to be relied upon, and this may not be adequate. It's also vital to realize that the body is healing – ultimately all healing is by the mind/body.

When talking to cancer survivors or reading their life stories, I have noticed their commitment to forestall the return of cancer or to control it. This becomes automatic for them. Eydie Mae Loeffler got off her program, ate quantities of sugar-laden dates and was soon fatigued. Small tumors in her breast enlarged almost overnight. She reversed course immediately and the tumors shrank back to what they had been. The foreboding event left her unfazed. Kay Bevan (given no chance to live ten years ago) matter-of-factly but cheerfully, said to me, *"Well, when you have cancer."* Anyone can take on this outlook – it could help save their life.

THE MECHANISM FOR HEALING

A small amount of shark cartilage helped one person, while another had to ingest greater amounts. The first woman may have hoped and expected that an exotic elixir such as shark cartilage would bring relief – *the puzzling placebo effect*. Though, Kay Bevan mentioned that some individuals with sensitive systems seem to do well with small amounts. Yet it still isn't fully known what shark cartilage actually does. Spontaneous remission for the deeply religious Catholic man supposes that the body is capable of overcoming cancer by itself (or with divine intervention). Other examples for curing cancer have been given. Albeit, none of this adequately explains how someone is actually cured. Nor is it truly understood why chemotherapy is sometimes effective.

All cells have a biological clock – everything in the universe may have an internal clock. Some cells of the human body live but a few hours, while others exist for many years. The body regulates this activity with precision. The ticking of the clock within cells may provide the answer for how cancer is eliminated. If it is true that cancer cells live longer than normal cells, it may be that treatments which are effective cause cancer cells to "speed up." In other words, not live as long as they have. Ultimately, cancer's ability to reproduce itself may be altered or interrupted. In a very recent study conducted on women with cancer of the cervix, an experimental treatment (not chemotherapy) stopped cancer cells from dividing. Tumors were quickly destroyed but normal tissue was unaffected.

A brief overview for successful alternative methods is this: in the beginning, cells of the immune system are immobilized or lethargic – the reason for cancer existing. Toxic sludge in the system is removed with cleansing techniques (enemas, colonics, juice fasting). This calms the body, eliminates inflammation and begins clearing the pancreas, liver, gallbladder and other organs. NK cells, white blood cells and the dendritic cells awaken. Nutritional supplements (Laetrile, germanium, Essiac, etc.) and proper food (organic grains and vegetables) rejuvenate the body. Additional accumulated cellular waste is purged, and the body is calmed even more.

Then, the command center orders the immune system to go on the offensive. The cells of the immune system are obsessed with killing cancer. It is what Nature intends of them. Even though cancer is a dimwitted abnormality, nevertheless, it is tenacious. If stress, poor digestion and bad health remain, cancer can succeed. Unwanted hormones and toxic sludge anesthetize the immune cells, confuse them and keep them from eradicating cancer. Dr. Gerson refers to *healing inflammation* which is necessary to reverse cancer. Remedies for cancer destroy cancer by penetrating its outer walls initially. However, for those who do survive cancer, the cells of the immune system unleash chemical warfare against cancer. They turn off or terminate cancer's ability to propagate itself. In reality, cancerous cells may not always be destroyed; they may remain as inactive defective cells.

MICROBES AND CANCER

Dr. Hulda Regehr Clark may be correct in believing parasites or microbes cause cancer. She provides case histories of those who were cured after they followed her recommendations. Dr. Clark forewarns that Black Walnut Hull tincture must be prepared and taken correctly if it is to be 100 percent effective. She suggests a seven day program whereby the amount of the tincture is increased gradually. According to Clark, known parasiticides (drugs) commonly prescribed throughout the world may not kill all stages of microbes, plus they are extremely toxic – not something to take if debilitated.

Clark adds that there must be dozens of plant derivatives (or methods) which destroy microbes. All vegetation (fruits, vegetables, trees) has defenses to contend with parasites or insects. The shell which protects the walnut is composed of bark, and wood has antibacterial properties. I learned DMSO is derived from wood. Vanillin, an artificial vanilla flavoring used in chocolate, is an extract from wood. Wine aged in wood caskets would have this ingredient.

Many cultures or societies use figs or castor bean oil to eliminate intestinal worms. What is in the skin of figs kills or sedates parasites. It is intriguing that figs are filled with seeds, while the castor bean is a seed. Someone said that deer eat bitter acorns at a certain time of the year. Parasites are killed and the digestive systems of the animals are coated and protected for months afterward. Onions are believed to kill bacteria, and germanium may also do this.

Dr. Gerson tells of witnessing "two cancers of the breast disappear with the use of fenugreek seeds tea in large amounts, combined with a saltless vegetarian diet." As a home remedy, crushed seeds of fenugreek are used as a poultice to remove warts – *abnormal growths attributable to a virus.* I'm certain fenugreek, if taken internally, would harm the immune systems for those of Blood Type B and Type AB.

Earlier, turmeric or curcumin (in curry) was said to have anti-cancer capabilities. Curry normally has additional herbs and spices. Fenugreek is frequently in curry, and at times, cardamom is included. Cardamom is antibacterial and may expunge parasites. Ginger, usually in curry, is known to expel worms. Japanese never eat raw fish without pickled ginger (and wasabi); the Chinese always add ginger when cooking fish and meats. Garlic, also in curry, rids bacteria and parasites. Black pepper kills bacteria and parasites. In fact, almost all of the herbs or spices in curries are antiinflammatory, antibacterial, anti-viral, antiparasitical or aid the immune system. Ancient herbalists realized this to some extent, but most people eating curried dishes today do so merely for the enjoyment of taste.

I said, in the Introduction, that I once followed macrobiotics. Three months after beginning the diet, a mole on my back festered, bled, crusted and fell off. This did concern me, but the problem passed within two days. Several months later, another mole on my back did the same thing; and then a gray mole on my shoulder came off as well. I believe organic brown rice in the macrobiotic diet was responsible for excising these superfluous growths. The brown rice (Laetrile and enzymes) is probably the underlying reason for the diet combating cancer.

Prior to the event with melanoma, I experienced severe hay fever, something I had never known in my life. Joints began to ache and my health deteriorated in strange ways, even hypoglycemia reappeared. Going back to total macrobiotics made no difference. Right up until the time of seeing the dermatologist, I was juggling diets, hoping something would help. Looking back, I can see that my immune system was malfunctioning badly. Knowing what I do now could have brought relief much earlier and better. And, just maybe, a potentially lethal skin cancer could have been avoided.

The story of a dog being cured of colon cancer with Black Walnut Hull tincture was mentioned. Since then, in a recent telephone conversation, I was told about a dog cured of cancer with some other underground remedy. In addition to these two examples, literature for The International Association of Cancer Victors and Friends lists a dog in Arkansas who it's said was cured of bone cancer with Laetrile, DMSO (presumably pharmaceutical grade and not the quality with aloe vera) and apricot kernels.

I wondered, if it was true, how could three dogs

have been cured of cancer? I decided to look to the dogs for an answer, not the remedies. I asked what characteristics or advantages might dogs have for surviving cancer when given a myriad of alternative remedies?

Dogs wouldn't be aware of how deadly the disease is. Emotional stress wouldn't be a problem and this would an advantage. Dogs are usually forgiving and seldom carry a grudge, and if in pain do their best to ignore it. These too would be advantages. Dogs know how to relax and get deep sleep – additional advantages for them. When in a home, dogs know their territory and are part of the "pack," and nurturing and petting are known to boost the immune system of animals. This gives them advantages. Dogs have extraordinary digestive systems and food passes quickly through their intestines, and any contaminated food is vomited effortlessly. These are other advantages. When sick, dogs stop eating, but once they recover instinctively eat what food is needed – another advantage for them. Having strong digestion may account for their powerful hormonal system which allows them to maintain superb muscle tone, even when merely stretching – definitely an advantage. Dogs are meat eaters and special diets are unnecessary – an advantage. Dogs can smell 200 times greater than humans and can detect plant medicines in a garden or yard quickly – maybe a big advantage. Once, after taken for a walk, our dog Sammie strained on his leash and refused to go into the house. After carefully inspecting dozens of plant shoots, he found the right one, chewed it with urgency and was at once satisfied. Dogs, being what they are, have distinct advantages and alternative medicines could possibly have complemented this enabling them to overcome cancer.

A conclusion: environmental contaminants from food or grass damage DNA of the dogs, and as a result nonfunctioning cells come into being. The dogs' immune system's ability to repair the body, fight disease or eliminate abnormal cells is undermined due to aging, damage to DNA or perhaps because of pollutants. The resulting inflammation from irritated tissue creates a habitat suitable for microbes introduced by fleas, mosquitoes, bed bugs, flies, food, or various larva in drinking water. One of the stages of development for microbes enters an abnormal cell – perhaps similar to the fertilization of an egg by sperm. DNA of the microbe or DNA from a toxin carried by the microbe helps transform the abnormal cell into cancer. The remedies described destroy both the cancerous cells and microbes. Laetrile and apricot kernels stimulate the immune system of the one dog to fight the disease or kill cancer cells. Mostly the dogs' own ability to relax in a deep way allows for healing.

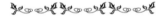

I had asked Dr. Gary Schwartz (associate professor of cancer biology at Wake Forest University) if parasites cause cancer. He said it was once believed they might. When viruses were discovered, the emphasis shifted to this. Toxins are now considered, but knowing what causes cancer is always ongoing, according to him. It is very possible that microbes are responsible for cancer.

CHAPTER TEN

Surviving Cancer

Most of the survivors I spoke with, received letters from, or read about indicated that at least some relaxation, rest or quiet time was included in their therapy. Notwithstanding this, it may be that deep relaxation (the example of the dogs) is the best method for healing the body and possibly surviving cancer. Yoga can provide this.

Yoga Instruction. Look in the *Yellow Pages*. *Yoga Today,* a monthly magazine available at book stores, is another source. Many health food stores have bulletin boards telling of yoga classes. (Being certified as an instructor has no significance.) Yogi Bhajan's 3HO kundalini yoga is easy to learn and extremely effective. I would advise anyone to receive instruction for this yoga at a 3HO center located in many cities throughout the country. "Intensives" are offered at the center in Española. This yoga can be done at home with books. Contact the organization for a catalog of its books, tapes and videos.

3HO/Ancient Healing Ways.
P.O. Box 130
Española, NM 87532
Tel: 800-359-2940.
Website: www.a-healing.com

These are some of the books offered: *Keeping Up With Kundalini Yoga; Yoga for Health, Relaxation & Well-Being; Kundalini Yoga: The Flow of Eternal Power; The Art, Science & Application of Kundalini Yoga.* Books contain photos and drawings of exercises. Meditations and breathing exercises are described. *"Breath of Fire"* may be as effective as some alternative oxygen therapies. The last book listed includes more than 40 sets and meditations. One set is to be done before sleeping at night. Kundalini yoga, if done fanatically or incorrectly, can release pent-up energies and cause serious physical or emotional problems. Hatha yoga, or another traditional form of yoga, may be safer and just as good. Improvised yoga would be dangerous!

YOGA EXPLAINED

Thousands of years ago, yogis (natural healers of India) noted the ailments which an agrarian-based society had brought and conceived the practice of yoga. Yoga consists of exercises for the body, the use of food as medicine, breathing routines and meditation. (Yogis knew long ago that eating too much protein causes senile dementia and also what is now named Alzheimer's.) Yoga is not a religion but many Asian religions often include it.

The exercise positions of yoga are known as postures and are named for animals. A group of postures is called a set. Each posture is arranged within the set for a distinct purpose. Sets have purposes too. For example, a posture or set may be intended to cleanse the kidneys, combat depression or elevate consciousness. The possibilities are considerable.

Performing a posture causes specific glands to secrete hormones. (Yogis advise against hormone replacement in most instances.) Usually there is a one minute rest after completing a posture, and during the rest, hormones flow throughout the body and are utilized by organs or other glands. Doing this keeps the body and immune system vibrant and balanced. Sexual fluids (produced from food), if allowed to mature, are absorbed by the spine and build nerves. The immune system is also strengthened.

Yoga is done early in the morning – 4:30 a.m. or before – everyday without exception. A brief chant – with palms of the hands together, thumbs tucked into the breast bone or heart center – focuses the mind and precedes the exercise routine. Chanting also invigorates the glands. Breathing exercises – some lasting for 15 minutes – follow the introductory chant. Necessary warm-up exercises are done after this. When each posture – usually for one to three minutes – is completed, a very deep inhale (through the nose) is taken and held for several seconds. The genital muscles are tightened, and on the forceful exhale, energy is circulated throughout the body, brought into the spine, then mentally released out the top of the skull. The body is relaxed at the same time.

When the lengthy set (not more than 45 minutes of physical exercise) ends, chanting may follow, but lying on the back is necessary soon after. For this, hands are at the side with palms facing up and the eyes are closed. A cloth to cover the eyes may be necessary if the room is not completely dark. A small towel rolled up and placed under the lower back or buttocks area can provide support. Breathing is very relaxed but long and deep – inhaling and exhaling through the nose.

A silent command for the toes to relax is given. Further mental suggestions to relax the soles of the feet, the ankles, shins, knees, legs, thighs, buttocks, stomach, fingers, hands, wrists, elbows, shoulders, neck, mouth, scalp, eyes, skull, nose and even eyebrows follow. The body melts onto the floor and the mind becomes detached. There are no thoughts – the past, future and present are dismissed. This deep relaxation lasts for at least 20 minutes. Some use a kitchen timer. During the relaxation, delta brain waves can often be felt "kicking in" or "rolling in." Sleep should be avoided. A white cotton blanket may be necessary for warmth.

After the rest, several extremely deep breaths are taken (always through the nose) and exhaled thoroughly, forcing out as much air as is comfortably possible. Consciousness is brought back and the feet and hands are shaken. Hands are rubbed together as are the feet. Turning over on one side and using the hands to rise prevents damage to the back.

With the eyes remaining closed, the lotus position of sitting is assumed — this for meditation, the ultimate goal of yoga. The legs are tucked under. Hands are placed on the knees, and deep but relaxed breathing continues. The eyes should be "seeing" out the forehead. Meditation is realizing the same delta brain waves when resting on the back. Most people have difficulty meditating. It is not simply sitting on the floor, closing the eyes and being quiet. Doing the complete routine of yoga, including the rest, are necessary for many. Meditation can be done for 20 minutes, but some forms of yoga encourage meditating for two and one half hours, or even meditating throughout the day whenever possible. Meditation at times, can produce "visions." Infrequently, hallucinations result. This usually isn't a problem. Fasting, not eating adequately, taking medications, and experiencing pain can also cause hallucinations.

Chanting can be part of meditation. Listening to tapes can provide this. The sound of rain falling in a tropical rain forest at night or an ocean washing against a shoreline could be excellent aids. The Aboriginal wind instrument, the didgeridoo, is able to take the mind into a trance and enhance meditation.

The silent meditation of Sa..Ta..Na..Ma will calm the mind. The "a" of the meditation is pronounced as "o" in top. This is repeated continuously. Each voiceless sound lasts a full second or four seconds total. This meditation and several which include the didgeridoo are available as tapes from 3HO. *New Age*, a publication available at new age shops and some health food stores, is also a source for unique tapes fitting for meditation. If playing tapes, the sound should be barely audible or very low. Gregorian chants could be effective. Many are addicted to some form of music – from popular to classical – and meditating to music which stimulates the brain is not advisable.

It is recommended that the spine be kept straight while meditating. For some, slumping the head and back just a bit works fine. Resting the back against a cushion is done by a few. Sitting on a hard surface is preferred to that of sitting on a soft couch. Putting pressure on the buttocks in this way releases stored fats and hormones.

Another objective of yoga is to perpetuate the pleasurable sensation – the releasing of endorphins – which meditation produces. Zen Buddhism refers to this as being in "the zone," while Charismatic Christians experience a mild version of "the Rapture." Wearing sunglasses continuously during the day will affect the brain's production of melatonin and adversely affect meditating and maintaining this sensation.

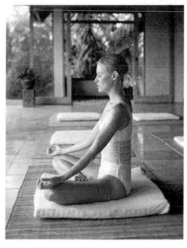

Buddhists believe that all unhappiness comes from having desires. For them, if all desires are eliminated, then one is on the path to enlightenment. Yoga advises not to dwell on possessions or positions. Being devoid of all desire for possessions or positions would put one on the path to tranquility, the goal for one intending to overcome a disease such as cancer.

Yoga is a method to change behavior. According to the Yogis, waking and meditating long before the sun rises allow the brain to secrete maximum melatonin. By exercising, chanting, meditating and deeply relaxing in the early hours of the morning consistently, self-control is gained. Being somewhat tired makes the brain more receptive to change, and meditation and deep relaxation easier to achieve. Yoga has no confidence in talk therapy unless the techniques and understanding of yoga are included. The Yogis also suggest fasting one day each week. This helps control cravings and overeating, and also enhances meditation and self-discipline.

When beginning yoga, stiffness and soreness are often experienced. If a particular exercise causes pain or problems, cease doing it. But gradually acclimating the body to stretching and breathing, and relaxing afterward, will usually deliver the desired results. With perseverance – making an honest effort but not pushing too hard – and patience, many are surprised at what they can accomplish. For yoga, it is important to keep the chin tucked in, the neck erect and "locked," and the spine straight. And never do headstands which some forms of yoga encourage.

Exercise programs other than yoga may not be helpful at all. I've known those who were unsuccessful in surviving cancer with a walking program. Obtain proper medical approval before doing any exercise routine, including yoga.

Natural opiates produced within the body through yoga and meditation may be preferable to painkillers. Taking narcotics (even marijuana) could possibly be harmful. Combining meditation with opium, morphine or another opiate can cause death. D'Adamo's plan suggests the supplement 5-HTP (a pleasant tranquilizer which quells fatigue and stress) for my blood type. It could help some to quit drinking and smoking. I find that a very tiny dash produces better results, but health food stores say many of their customers require one or two capsules. Whether this supplement – derived from an obscure seed – would be helpful or not for those diagnosed with cancer isn't known. Refer to D'Adamo's books for what may be helpful for your blood type.

SOLITUDE

Minimizing stimulus to the senses is a yoga concept and may be needed in extreme situations. Television, radio and any music – except chanting – would be turned off. No reading would be done. There would be no talking whatsoever; all communication would be through written messages. There would be no emotional upheavals. No anger. No sadness. One would be content and maintain an inner glow. Any humor recalled would be enjoyed in total silence.

Correct sleep is crucial. One would go to bed extremely early in the evening. Lying on the floor and lifting both legs and pointing the soles of feet toward the ceiling is a yoga technique to deepen sleep. Yogis do this for 15 minutes prior to sleeping at night – novices often place their legs against a wall. When doing this, the buttocks must touch the wall and a small rolled up towel should be place under the neck. Stretching exercises and relaxed breathing would be done before sleep as well. Yogis advise abstaining from sexual intercourse; avoiding sex would enhance relaxation and meditation.

Sleeping on a futon (a thick cotton-filled mattress laid on the floor) is preferred by some. A Swedish Dux™ bed may be a good choice, but a thin pad may even be better. However, sleeping on pads may be too difficult for some. Yoga Mats in San Francisco offers pads. For a catalog for mats, pads, bolsters and Shoji screens (folding room dividers), contact the company. Tel: 800-720-YOGA.

The room slept in would be completely white. Shoji screens would do, but white sheets could be tacked to the walls. Large rugs or carpeted areas would be covered with white sheets. Sheets, blankets, loosely worn clothing and long nightclothing – both fresh and clean every day – would be of pure white cotton. Clothes would be washed with non-perfumed soap powder, and clothing slept in would not be worn when exercising or at other times. A small white cotton rug or yoga pad would provide a place to practice yoga and meditate. Objects not white would be removed, but some green plants would be allowed. For Yogis nothing is more healing that white – the reason for hospitals being white, though this has been forgotten.

Battery-powered camping lamps and flashlights would provide light at night or in the morning. Trash containers with garbage would not be allowed to remain in the house to pollute the air. If the house is sealed tight, the air would be toxic. Breathing fresh air – not cold air – would be better. It would be wise to follow Dr. Hulda Regehr Clark's advice and know that the environment (and body) is free of contaminants which may be contributing to cancer or affecting the immune system – refer to her books.

Caring for the body. A mild daily self-massage would be beneficial. Gently rubbing the feet every day would help eliminate the sensation of "tiny crystals" embedded under the skin. Pressing the feet against rough rocks in a cat box, even if seated, would do this, and would be sedating as well. Paying for a full body massage could be considered. Sponge baths in the morning and before bed with distilled water – never allow the body to become chilled – would be a daily routine. Yogis take ice-cold showers before exercising, but not when ill. No metal would touch the skin. Chemicals of any kind would be avoided. No coloring agents or permanent solutions would be applied to the hair. Gerson says not to brush the teeth with bicarbonate of soda or baking soda. Tea would be made and drunk in the manner of the Japanese – a lengthy ornate ceremony where quiet and calm are emphasized.

Yoga exercises in the early hours of the day would be a daily ritual. Other exercise during the day would be limited to stretching and light workouts. Resting on the back (or stomach) in the afternoon for the recommended time would be permissible. Chanting and meditation can be done in the evening for an hour or longer.

Yogis say the body should take more energy from breathing air than from eating food. Breathing correctly throughout the day would be an objective. One exercise for breathing is to sit and breathe long and deep in a slow manner for 30 minutes or more at a time. Upon waking in the morning, adrenaline floods the body. Some Yogis immediately sit on the floor and begin long, deep breathing, or chanting. But the full yoga routine is suggested.

Yogi Bhajan said, "Death is nothing more than a good sleep." Traditionally, Yogis long to reunite with their Creator. This thought is comforting to them. Anyone can draw upon their own faith to be consoled. This can be done as a silent affirmation within the concept of solitude.

If waking early from panic attacks or stress, Yogis advise not to remain in bed and suffer but immediately begin stretching exercises on the floor. One exercise is to sit on the floor, tuck the heel of the right foot into the groin area, then stretch down over the extended left leg. The toe is grasped with the left hand – the thumb is pressed onto the bottom of the big toe. The right hand squeezes the sole of the left foot. If possible, the head touches the knee. One relaxes down into the position and continues with long, slow but deep inhales and exhales. The extended leg should be flat on the ground. The position can be reversed for the other leg. Within 10 minutes, the crisis should pass. If someone is overweight or isn't agile and cannot stretch over their extended leg, they shouldn't be discouraged. Keeping the leg flat on the floor and extending the head over will suffice. Continue to relax without doing any harm.

The 3HO Yogis wrap their heads tightly in turbans for the entire day, even while sleeping. Covering the head when meditating or exercising is advised; most heat of the body is lost through the skull. A ski cap, hood or shawl will do. Keeping the body and head warm at all times is a good health practice. This may be necessary for the time of solitude.

CHAPTER ELEVEN

Afterthoughts

A young assertive female executive in a high-pressure position spoke of her recurrence of breast cancer. She described her "healthy" lifestyle of doing hard workouts for several hours each day, and took pride in saying she had been a vegetarian for much of her life – she was stir-frying vegetables in a wok inundated with an unknown vegetable oil.

Attacking work as this young woman did could have created an imbalance for her hormones leading to cancer. Though, exercising in the manner she did and not relaxing afterward could have contributed. Despite these possibilities, the vegetable oil could be a cause. It was heated to high temperatures; it may have been incorrect for her blood type; it may have contained solvents or toxins; and, the quantity of oil consumed by her was far more than what is appropriate for anyone's diet. Fats in the body interact with hormones and cells could have become cancerous because of this oil. Dr. Budwig (the advocate of flaxseed) may say this is exactly what occurred. Possibly following D'Adamo's plan, changing her lifestyle, and including yoga and deep relaxation in her daily activity would help return good health to this woman. The relaxation described must be genuine and profound – self-deception could prove fateful.

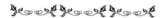

Some have found D'Adamo's plan too difficult, while others will not accept it. Even Dr. D'Adamo doesn't follow his plan totally. Most would benefit with the plan, however food allergies or food sensitivities may remain. And not all foods considered beneficial will become favorites. People are creatures of habit and culture and have conditioned their bodies to foods which they should not be eating. I had great difficulty giving up bread and grains but finally did. I adapted to the plan by eating those foods which were agreeable, and others were introduced slowly. However, foods and supplements beneficial for non-secretors of my blood type are very necessary; only these keep me at my best.

In the past I have had high blood pressure, periodically rising to levels of alarm. Usually, I would alter my diet, exercise more, drink vegetable juices, miss a meal or go to bed early and this would solve the problem. In recent years this hasn't always worked. Having a blood type known for "constantly starving" doesn't help, but my blood pressure is normal now. Recently during a holiday, I got off the plan, ate Mexican food, drank wine and included other abuses. My blood pressure skyrocketed. Returning to appropriate foods soon ended that. This doesn't mean that I never cheat on the plan.

Mild but chronic lower back pain is gone. I've never

exercised better in my life. I maintain good muscle tone. I sleep terrifically – not so when I was on a grain/vegetarian diet. Meditation is extremely easy. Doing simple tasks before often created anxiety; now I am calm and eager for most anything. Also, my immune system has never been better. I see evidence for this every day.

Having cold hands and being exceptionally cold in winter for a lifetime are greatly diminished now. I've come to enjoy cold weather. In East Asia, it's a sign of good health when the body is able to generate heat naturally. Eating dogs in winter is common in East Asia. Dogs are carnivores and their flesh is saturated with uric acid. Such meat produces internal heat when eaten, but it's clear why humans throughout the world rarely eat animals which eat meat. Yogis believe pranic energy (heat created from exercise and meditation) will "burn up" disease. Exercises which flex the spine are noted for producing this heat. There are those in India who bury themselves in snow and use meditation alone to generate pranic heat to melt the ice enclosing them. They stage contests to see who is fastest to free himself.

On several occasions I have eaten beef, mutton or chicken which I purchased at a grocery store or ordered at a restaurant. In every case – even when eating pure red cube steaks termed natural – I awoke early from not sleeping well and soon began spitting and coughing a nasty phlegm. This went on all morning and part of the afternoon. When cooking bison or grass-fed beef in a small amount of water, there is never any leftover fat (or very little) in the pan, nor do these meats taste fatty. And phlegm never accumulates in my throat later. I once bought rabbit which appeared lean but was filled with fat. Wild rabbits which I shot and ate many decades ago tasted great. It is evident rabbits sold at markets are either fed grain or given feed which is questionable.

It's usually recommended that meat be thoroughly cooked to kill any bacteria. However, to get the full benefit (and enzymes), meat should be cooked somewhat rare. D'Adamo suggests this, and I discovered it to be true. Unfortunately, I have research (nasty photos) which shows all the parasites and microbes in meat. So, what can be done? Buy meat from a market which at least appears to be carrying out good health practices. Eat onions and other foods known to be antimicrobial. Good digestion is essential – take the correct digestive aids for your blood type if need be. Eat the foods indicated in the plan. Eat less. Stay active. That's all anyone can do.

Massage therapy was recommended earlier. I took my own advice and asked the masseuse not to hold back – she didn't. I had forgotten what a hard elbow pressed up and down the spine for 15 minutes can do. I felt terrific but was lightheaded. This made meditating easy. Massage therapy is often used to treat pain, and for some individuals may make painkillers unnecessary or less required.

Someone I know recently began D'Adamo's plan and in a brief time went from weighing almost 200 pounds to weighing 165. He said he isn't eating less and that he feels better. His older brother had surgery for prostate cancer and there is the possibility my friend may have a problem now. A biopsy is being considered but he may do nothing. Prostate cancer may soon be detectable by analyzing a single drop of blood, making biopsies unnecessary. This individual is Blood Type AB, and I told him that he should be eating snails once every week or so.

It may be that only following the plan (D'Adamo's research for foods and substances are limited but adequate) would lower the odds for developing cancer from one in four to one in 12. And, that if a healthy lifestyle is introduced, the odds could be extended to one in 40. One in eight women develops breast cancer. Perhaps these odds could be increased to one in 64, or even greater. Avoiding cancer would make life better for everyone.

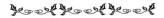

The people in Iceland are predominately Type O. The majority are descendants of those who sailed a millennium ago from Norway which is my ancestry. Icelanders are highly literate, industrious and prosperous. The ocean which surrounds them provides numerous fish beneficial for their blood type. They do not have soil or climate suitable for growing grains but grains aren't required anyway. With greenhouses – heat is supplied from an underground source – adequate vegetables can be grown. It should not be surprising they do well. They do have some problem with alcoholism, and perhaps with depression due to lack of sunlight at times. But chronic fatigue, hyperactivity, attention deficit disorder, obesity in children and rampant antisocial behavior (one in 32 in America is now in prison or in the criminal justice system) are not problems for them, from what I know. The cold weather would help to keep them physically active. If not, lack of exercise would increase their risk for cancer. Consuming processed foods – fast foods imported from America – would do this as well.

Icelanders hang shark meat in sheds for curing and the flesh develops a heavy mold. This delicacy could well be carcinogenic. Literature sent by Dr. Gary Schwartz included studies which showed that during World War II, rates of testicular cancer dropped dramatically throughout Scandinavia. During this time, food was limited and pork, shark or processed foods were not available. Since World War II, testicular cancer has increased steadily every year in the entire region. Growing affluence since that time has allowed greater access for processed foods and incidents for all cancer are on the rise. Many Icelanders enjoy steam baths and mud baths, and others in Scandinavia take to saunas, and this may rid their bodies of some dangerous toxins. I would recommend D'Adamo's diet plan to them and suggest they avoid foods known to contribute to cancer.

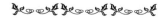

Developed to remove deadly uranium from survivors of the Chernobyl disaster, **Modifilan**, derived from brown seaweed (*Laminaria japonica*), was found to also detoxify the body of heavy metals and other toxins. Research supplied by the company's director Sergei Zimin indicates Modifilan may be effective in the treatment of cancer. Pacific Standard Distributors, Inc., states its product has been prepared with unique low temperature technology which makes its raw seaweed extract safe and very digestible. To produce one pound of Modifilan requires 40 pounds of brown seaweed – it is not simply seaweed. Though the company recommends greater amounts for certain conditions, lesser amounts may be prudent initially. Modifilan is be taken on an entirely empty stomach – never with food. See its Website: www.modifilan.com or Tel: 650-853-1131. Zimin anticipates Modifilan will soon be available in health food stores.

In the Chapter for Alternative Remedies, I didn't list all of the methods which are known. The books I commented upon in the Introduction mention others. If you do further research, you will discover more. Three individuals interviewed on television several years ago claimed to have been cured of cancer with natural remedies I don't recall. One said that when cancer was put into remission, his doctor attributed it to a delayed reaction from the chemotherapy. The individual corrected him saying chemotherapy had nothing to do with it.

The Associate Press reported on a new alternative method called anti-angiogenics. It differs from chemotherapy in that blood vessels which feed tumors are targeted, not the tumors themselves. Most studies had been disappointing until Sugen (www.sugen.com) developed a drug which shrank tumors by more than 50 percent in six of 23 mostly terminal patients. Reduction was for a variety of tumors. Researchers were surprised and delighted – no one knows if anyone will actually be cured.

A segment of a recent *60 Minutes* program was about a young father terminal with cancer. With nothing to lose, he was allowed to be tested in a trial. Four times the usual amount of a known chemotherapy were injected into his body. The cancer was soon gone. Quite likely, thousands of cancer patients watching the show will now ask to receive similar treatment. Physicians know that most would die from this treatment.

A local television station mentioned that a notable medical clinic in Texas will soon begin testing shark cartilage and wheat grass juice as possible treatments for cancer. The pharmaceutical companies will be watching closely. I fully expect the clinic's study to eventually declare that neither shark cartilage nor wheat grass juice offers any promise in the treatment of cancer.

The health commentator (also a physician) for another television station reported on the findings of a medical journal which said colon cancer results from red meat and processed foods intensifying cell growth in the lining of the colon. In some enigmatic way, evidently, cancer cells then come into being. The medical journal and the television commentator were ignoring the statistical documentation already collected on cancer and blood types. They are also unacquainted with research showing the link between cancer and microbes.

⁕⁕⁕

I indicated earlier that Chinese medicine includes acupressure in healing. Acupressure (also known as pressure point therapy) is used for just about every common ailment. Books on acupressure say it is not a therapy for cancer but is suitable for combating stress, promoting good sleep, and building the immune system. For this therapy, pressure is applied on a particular part of the body with a thumb, a finger or several fingers, and is maintained for up to several minutes. This is a treatment for constipation: while lying down, a thumb is pressed onto the stomach in six or seven places circularly around the stomach. Pressure is maintained at each point for up to three minutes.

I have concluded that dogs sleeping on hard ground or pavement are stimulating their immune systems with pressure point therapy. This would be the same for humans sleeping on hard surfaces. It also occurred to me that yoga has elements of acupressure. Sitting on the floor for meditation is pressure point therapy as is any stretching. One yoga posture (standing with hands resting on the knees) involves forcefully exhaling all air, sucking in the stomach to where it almost touches the spine, then lifting the diaphragm. Yogis say that doing this twice each day will prevent colon or stomach cancer.

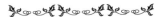

Stephanie Nano wrote this for The Associated Press: *The New England Journal of Medicine* recently reported that two individuals in Scotland developed melanoma cancer after receiving transplanted kidneys from a donor who had a melanoma skin lesion removed 16 years earlier. He was thought to be cancer-free. One patient has since died, while the other is said to have recovered. According to Nano's article, the melanoma cells apparently had been dormant in the kidneys until the transplant. When medicines to prevent organ rejection were injected, cancer cells were activated as the immune system was suppressed. Someone told me she had a friend who also received a kidney transplant and developed cancer. Her donor was unaware that he had the disease. These are good examples of how important the immune system is in preventing and overcoming cancer.

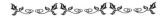

A few days before sending my files for printing, I was fortunate to acquire Jason Winters' book *Killing*

Cancer – an edition printed in 1983. In the late 1970s, doctors told Winters he would die from the rapidly growing cancerous tumor in his neck. Refusing to be mutilated by surgery and radiation, he went to Mexico for Laetrile therapy. The tumor went down in size, but soon enlarged again. Winters then flew to Singapore for an exotic herbal remedy – which also didn't work. A trip to Tibet was made later. Eventually, Winters created Tribalene which consists of four herbs – one being red clover. Other herbs included were a mix of beneficials, neutrals or avoids for each of the four blood types; but all blood types are to avoid red clover, according to D'Adamo. Jason Winters markets Tribalene at health food stores – no claims are made. His book is a fascinating account of what he did to survive. To my knowledge he is alive today.

LAST MINUTE ADDENDUM

Stopping by the library at press deadline, I discovered the *American Cancer Society's Guide to Complementary and Alternative Cancer Methods*. I was unaware that the book existed, even though I had spoken to the Society previously. Every possible alternative remedy is discussed in some detail.

RESOURCES

ASSOCIATIONS:
The International Association of Cancer Victors and Friends, Inc. (non-profit organization)
7740 West Manchester Ave., Suite 203
Playa del Rey, CA 90293
Tel: 310-822-5032, 310-822-4593..

Cancer Victors Journal is its quarterly publication. The IACVF lists 100 cancer survivors who may be contacted by telephone or mail. Survivors state what type of cancer they had, where they were treated, and the treatments they received. Membership dues are $25. Cancer Doctor: The Biography of Josef Issels, M.D., by Gordon Thomas and Cancer: A Second Opinion by Josef Issels can be ordered directly. Issels treated (with vaccines) more than 12,000 cancer patients who had been written off as "incurable" by other doctors. One Answer to Cancer by Carol Morrison-Kelley, M.D., is another book available from the IACVF.

World Research Foundation (non-profit organization)
41 Bell Rock Plaza
Sedona, AZ 86351
Tel: 520-284-3300.

> *Research for almost every ailment including cancer – everything from bladder cancer, breast cancer to uterine cancer – is offered. Over 25,000 medical journals and several hundred thousand data banks are accessed. Reports cost about $70. A donation is requested for membership.*

People Against Cancer (non-profit organization)
604 East St., PO Box 10
Otho, IA 50569
Tel: 515-972-4444.

> *Information on alternative therapy is offered. Many who work here are volunteers; some are cancer survivors or have had a family member who died from cancer. Request current fees.*

Foundation for Advancement in Cancer Therapy (non-profit organization)
Box 1242, Old Chelsea Station
New York, NY 10113
Tel: 212-741-2790.

> *Information for prevention of cancer and alternative methods of treatment are provided. Call or write for current price list. Include a SASE if writing. A donation is requested. Books, publications and tapes of personal histories of recovered cancer patients are offered. Some survivors – told they were terminally ill – have remained alive and healthy for more than 40 years.*

Life Extension
P.O. Box 229120
Hollywood, FL 33022
el: 800-841-5433.

*Extensive research on all health problems is pro-
vided by the organization. The March 2002 edition of Life Extension (its magazine) included an
article about melatonin as a treatment for cancer.
The July 2002 edition reported that theanine (an
amino acid extracted form tea) enhances chemotherapy by overcoming cancer's ability to resist
it. Another article, in the July 2002 edition, titled
"Prostate Cancer Success" described how an elderly man was cured of prostate cancer with drugs,
not radiation. Other articles within were: "A Report On Curcumin's Anti-Cancer Effects." and
"Silibinin: The Better Form of Silymarin." More
recent editions discussed tocotrienols for treating breast cancer, and lycopene. Also, Cimetidine
(Tagamet™) may put cancer in remission.*

CLINICS:

Livingston Foundation Medical Center
3232 Duke St.
San Diego, CA 92110
Tel: 619-224-3515, 888-777-7321

*The Center was founded in 1970 by the late Dr.
Virginia C. Livingston who believed that a cure
for cancer could be realized through the body's
immune system. Part of the Livingston program
consists of six vaccines, most patented by
Livingston. The Cancer Microbe by Alan
Cantwell, Jr., M.D., and The Conquest of Cancer
written by Dr. Livingston can be ordered from
the foundation. Request brochures.*

BOOKS:

Third Opinion by John M. Fink.
This is a directory of medical centers which treat cancer and other degenerative diseases with alternative methods. Addresses, phone numbers, methods of treatments and costs for several hundred facilities located all over the world are included.

Questioning Chemotherapy by Ralph W. Moss, Ph.D.
Chemotherapy damages the immune system and alternative methods of treatment should be considered. Dr. Moss has written numerous books on cancer.

Free Your Body of Tumors and Cysts by Rev. Hanna Kroeger, Ms.D.
Her research may be of benefit.

The Complete Encyclopedia of Natural Healing by Gary Null, Ph.D.
More than 50 cancer patients, many terminal, give details of their experiences in surviving. Homeopathy, oxygen therapy, Qi Gong, 714-X, and the Gerson Diet are some treatments discussed. Information about clinics in Mexico and doctors licensed to practice in the United States is included.

Heinerman's Encyclopedia of Healing Juices by John Heinerman.
Beet juice may keep one from cancer. Wheat grass and barley grass juices – "A Renewal of Life in Every Glass."

Prevention

The monthly health publication regularly includes articles on cancer prevention. The August 2002 edition featured a story titled "Nothing Left to Lose" which told of four cancer patients – three terminal – who turned to alternative treatments many years ago and remain cancer-free today.

Mother Earth News

Lots of good health information in this monthly magazine available at newsstands. In the April/May 2002 edition, an article titled "Perfect Pasture" told of benefits of grass-fed meats. The author recommended visiting eatwild.com.

Alternative Medicine

Numerous articles about alternative treatments for cancer. Life stories, sources, books and places. Available at health food stores.

NEWSLETTERS:

Prescriptions for Healthy Living

James F. Balch, M.D., renowned co-author of Prescription for Nutritional Healing, the world's number one best-selling book on drug-free healing, offers advice for safer medicines. Tel: 800-728-2288.

Second Opinion

Dr. Robert J. Rowen, Phi Beta Kappa graduate of Johns Hopkins University, pioneered the nation's first statutory protection for alternative medicine in 1990. Rowen publishes an excellent health newsletter. Tel: 800-728-2288.

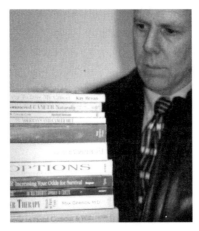

NOTES